The Wonder and the Mystery: 10 Years of Reflections from the *Annals of Family Medicine*

Edited by

ROBIN S. GOTLER

Reflections Editor
Annals of Family Medicine

Foreword by

RACHEL NAOMI REMEN
MD

Radcliffe Publishing
London • New York

Radcliffe Publishing Ltd
33–41 Dallington Street
London
EC1V 0BB
United Kingdom

www.radcliffehealth.com

———————————————————————

British Library Cataloguing in Publication Data

A catalogue record for this book is available from the British Library.

ISBN-13: 978 184619 982 0

Typeset by Darkriver Design, Auckland, New Zealand
Printed and bound by Cadmus Communications, USA

Contents

Contents

Contents

Contents

Foreword

Some Thoughts on Mystery and Wonder

Wonder is not an idea; it is an experience, the natural response to being in the presence of something larger and more universal than ourselves. There is a great deal in medicine that is worthy of wonder and awe. We witness acts of courage and commitment, of love, compassion, generosity, and sacrifice. There are moments when we are confronted with the power of faith or the will to live in all of its many manifestations or ordinary people in dark times rising above themselves to become all that they can be. We witness the power of healing. Yet very little in our training prepares us to notice the experiences of wonder and awe that occur in our everyday work.

Primary care is a natural setting for wonder; it has always been more than a set of medical techniques and skills. Caring for whole people and their families, their grandparents and their grandchildren, often includes aspects not covered in our professional training, dimensions that cannot be measured or replicated but only experienced. The authors in this book reveal primary care in all its fullness and complexity, each from their own unique perspective. Some speak of love and relationship; others, about new systems that can better serve whole people and their communities; still others, about the deep and universal meaning of this work. Many share stories of intimacy, commitment, and deep caring. They remind us that we have chosen this work not because of the science but because of the people.

When we become open to seeing people as well as their problems, we invite wonder and even mystery into our examining rooms. We reclaim our work as an opportunity to go beyond the ordinary in human relationships and witness the full range of human responses and capacities. What we see and hear may raise questions we have not asked ourselves before, questions we may not have even recognized as relevant to medicine. Caring for whole people may cause us to wonder as well as to diagnose and treat, and, in doing so, to discover inspiration and renewal.

An emergency room physician once told me about something that happened on an ordinary night in the emergency room. In the midst of a busy shift he had been called STAT to see a woman in active labor brought in by ambulance. A quick examination in the ambulance bay while she was still on a gurney told him that the birth was imminent. It was doubtful that her obstetrician would arrive in time to deliver and so he spoke to the woman, telling her that he had delivered many babies in the emergency room and if her baby arrived before her doctor, he would deliver her himself. He had barely finished reassuring her when the birth began in earnest. With an emergency room nurse and a paramedic on either side of him holding the mother's legs on their shoulders, Harry successfully delivered her of a baby girl. Despite the strangeness of the surroundings, the birth had gone perfectly and Harry experienced a familiar sense of pride in his own skills and competency. Holding the infant along his forearm he had lowered her below the placenta and had just begun to suction her nose and mouth when suddenly she opened her eyes and looked directly at him. There was an expression of wonder on her face. In that moment, Harry stepped past his usual way of seeing things and realized something astonishing; he was the first human being that this infant had ever seen. He felt his heart go out to her in welcome and for a brief moment there were tears in his eyes. This surprised him but it did not render him incompetent and he completed the delivery and handed the baby off to the pediatric resident as usual. However, Harry says he feels changed by this experience. In the moment when the infant opened her eyes, he felt years of cynicism and depression fall away from him and was flooded with an unfamiliar feeling. It took him 2 days to identify what it was but eventually he realized that the feeling was gratitude for being the one who got to stand there on the threshold of the world and welcome her. He smiles and says perhaps she was the first baby he had ever really delivered. In the past he would have been there only as a physician and not as a human being. As a physician, he might not have noticed the baby open her eyes or realized what her look had meant. Harry is not a poetic guy but he refers to the moment when the baby looked into his eyes as a "holy moment." He wonders how many such moments of awe and renewal he has missed in his many years in the emergency room. He suspects there have been many. So he looks for them on purpose now and he finds them everywhere.

Much can blind us to the experiences of wonder that are a part of our work. We can become focused on specific tasks or goals or deadlines, weighted down by committee meetings and paper work, frustrated and exasperated by regulations and the many difficulties we encounter daily. We can become so self-protective that we do not get close enough to others to see what is awesome in them and their stories, or cynical enough that we may have even forgotten how to see.

Perhaps all that is needed to find renewal and inspiration in our work is to begin to see the familiar in new ways. We may need to step beyond the perspective of our expertise for a moment and become more than we have been trained to be, to recognize that the elegance with which science describes life does not completely define life. That life is larger than our science, larger than our theories, larger than ourselves. That it is possible to research life for years without knowing life at all.

Years ago during an in-service for physicians on finding the meaning in our work, one of us suggested that we all take out our stethoscopes and listen to our own hearts for 7 minutes. Not wishing to embarrass her by refusing this odd request, we all complied. We were a group of middle-aged people and looking around me I saw expressions of concern on several faces. Was that an opening click? A gallop? A third heart sound? But 7 minutes is actually a rather long time and slowly we passed through this period of anxiety and intellect into something completely different, something far beyond the ordinary; a sort of meditation on the life force itself. We were all deeply moved by it and after a long silence we discussed this experience at length. The first to speak was the only cardiologist among us who simply said, "I have auscultated thousands of hearts but I have never heard a single one."

Our work presents us not only with experiences of wonder and awe but also with experiences of mystery. We all have our stories and the sort of questions whose answers cannot be found in any medical textbook.

My first experience of mystery in medicine happened when I was a very new intern. At 3:00 one morning when I was on call for pediatrics, a mother brought her 18-month-old to the hospital in a state of panic. "There is something terribly wrong with my baby," she told the front desk. "My baby is going to die." Awakened by a hand on my shoulder I stumbled into an examining room to hear her frantic story. She had been in bed asleep only a short time ago and awoke filled with dread and the certainty that her child was in danger. I looked at the little boy. He giggled and reached out to me with both hands. Carefully I went over him but found nothing. His breathing was perhaps a little too fast and he had half a degree of fever. I ordered a chest X-ray, a urinalysis, and a complete blood count. All normal. I sat down to share these findings with his mother but she was not reassured. She became even more anxious and insistent that her baby was in danger. Meanwhile, the little boy explored the room, opening drawers and trying to climb on each of the chairs. Baffled, I called my resident to present the case and ask about the possibility of doing a lumbar puncture. He was outraged. "Send her home," he told me, his voice dripping scorn. Chastened, I went back to the examining room to tell her the news. Hearing it, she burst into tears. Despite the absence of findings, I was impressed with the intensity of her fear. Hesitantly, I asked if she would give me permission to do a lumbar puncture. Without hesitation she agreed.

The nurses looked askance when I asked for assistance and a set up, but they complied. With their help and the help of the baby's mother, I began the procedure. I had just felt the needle snap through the dura when the door to the examining room burst open. There was my resident, his face red with anger. But I was already in deep trouble and so I pressed on. With a shaking hand I pulled the stylet from the needle. Nothing. "What are you doing?" my resident shouted, and holding the needle steady against the baby's back I turned to answer him. Suddenly his glance slid past my face to my hands. I turned my head just in time to see the first drop of pus fall from the needle. Pneumococcal meningitis. Unless rapidly treated, a cause of brain damage, deafness, epilepsy, even death.

Silently my resident helped me start an IV, take cultures, begin treatment, and admit the child. Afterward he clapped me on the shoulder. "Nice pick-up," he said to me. "Good thing you noticed that rapid respiration rate." But of course that was not the reason I had defied his orders. I have never found a medical explanation for this story, but I carry the memory of it with me and occasionally it saves someone's life.

We have all encountered more mystery and wonder than we have allowed to touch us, awaken us, or inspire us. The culture of medicine does not help us cultivate a sense of comfort with things that cannot be measured. Indeed, anything not evidence based may even be seen as not real. The search for certainty and control that dominates our medical culture and our thinking may have impoverished our lives. We have traded mystery for mastery, but only at a great price. As a profession we have lost a sense of wonder, of awe, of aliveness, and we have traded it for numbness, cynicism, depression, and compassion fatigue.

Wonder, awe, and mystery have become a part of the Shadow of our highly technical lives. Jung defines Shadow as those aspects of our personal wholeness and life's wholeness that are collectively denied, disavowed, and thrust out of daily awareness. It takes a sort of courage to re-own aspects of the Shadow. It may require letting go of our usual way of seeing things, and our pride in knowing things, and becoming willing to simply wonder together. But the rewards are great. People who wonder rarely burn out.

The things we cannot measure may be the very things that will sustain us, that form the foundation of a life of service and deep fulfillment. Primary care is not just a work of science; primary care is a front row seat on life, a rare glimpse of the wonder and mystery present below the surface of the ordinary, invisible to the casual observer. We may all need to know a little less and wonder a little more. *The Wonder and the Mystery: 10 Years of Reflections from the* Annals of Family Medicine offers us a powerful reminder to do this.

Rachel Naomi Remen, MD
January 2013

About the Editor

Robin S. Gotler, MA, is Reflections Editor of the *Annals of Family Medicine*. She received a Bachelor of Arts degree in Philosophy and Sociology of Health and Disease from the College of St. Catherine and Master of Arts degrees in Bioethics (Case Western Reserve University) and History of Medicine (University of Minnesota). She has a passion for essays and memoir, nurtured by her studies of creative nonfiction with Carol Bly and Catherine Watson in the woods of northern Minnesota. Robin has been privileged to work in family medicine for 25 years and with the *Annals of Family Medicine* since its inception in 2002. She lives with her family in Minnesota, where wonder and mystery abound.

Contributors

Richard E. Allen, MD, MPH, is the Residency Program Director at St. Mark's Family Medicine in Salt Lake City, Utah.

Steve M. Blevins, MD, is Associate Professor of Medicine and Assistant Dean for Curriculum Development at the University of Oklahoma Health Sciences Center.

Thomas Bodenheimer, MD, MPH, has practiced full-time primary care medicine for 32 years.

Jeffrey Borkan, MD, PhD, is a family physician-medical anthropologist who combines clinical work, education, research, and advocacy into his roles as Professor and Chair of the Department of Family Medicine, Brown University.

Howard Brody, MD, PhD, is the John P. McGovern Centennial Chair in Family Medicine and Director of the Institute for the Medical Humanities at the University of Texas Medical Branch in Galveston.

Lucy M. Candib, MD, is an author who practices and teaches family medicine, including obstetrics, at a community health center serving a multiethnic population in Worcester, Massachusetts.

Joseph A. Carrese, MD, MPH, is a general internist/primary care physician, as well as Associate Professor of Medicine and core faculty member at the Berman Institute of Bioethics, Johns Hopkins University.

Ellen Chen, MD, is a family physician and the Medical Director of the Silver Avenue Family Health Center in San Francisco, California.

Ian Douglas Couper, BA, MBBCh, MFamMed, is a family physician in the North West province Department of Health, South Africa, and Director of the University of the Witwatersrand Centre for Rural Health.

Patrick Crommett, now deceased, was a principal dancer with the Royal Swedish Ballet and later moved to his family homestead near Batesville, Arkansas, where he taught dance to children and choreographed community theater productions.

Thomas R. Egnew, EdD, LICSW, is the Behavioral Science Coordinator at Tacoma Family Medicine, Tacoma, Washington, and a Clinical Professor in the Department of Family Medicine, University of Washington School of Medicine, Seattle, Washington.

Contributors

Zachary Flake, MD, is a family physician at Columbine Family Practice in Loveland, Colorado.

John J. Frey III, MD, finished his residency in 1973 and has practiced and taught since then, learning family medicine from his patients and colleagues. He works in Madison, Wisconsin.

Dean Gianakos, MD, is a family medicine and medical humanities teacher in the Lynchburg Family Medicine Residency and Geriatrics Fellowship Program, Lynchburg, Virginia.

James L. Glazer, MD, FACSM, is a family physician, sports medicine specialist, and author in southern Maine.

Cherie Glazner, MD, MSPH, practices and teaches full-spectrum family medicine in Colorado when she is not outside gardening or riding her bike in the mountains.

Larry A. Green, MD, is Professor of Family Medicine and the Epperson Zorn Chair for Innovation in Family Medicine and Primary Care at the University of Colorado Denver.

Paul Haidet, MD, MPH, is a general internist, health services and education researcher, and jazz enthusiast at the Pennsylvania State University College of Medicine. He is a past president of the American Academy on Communication in Healthcare.

Hali Hammer, MD, is a family physician and Medical Director of the San Francisco General Hospital Family Health Center and an Associate Director of the University of California, San Francisco–San Francisco General Hospital Family and Community Medicine Residency Program.

Leif Hass, MD, is a family medicine physician who leads the Alta Bates Summit Medical Center Hospital Medicine Program in Oakland, California, and serves as a mentor for the Clinical Excellence Research Center at Stanford University.

Michel A. Ibrahim, MD, PhD, is Professor of Epidemiology and Editor-in-Chief of *Epidemiologic Reviews*, Johns Hopkins Bloomberg School of Public Health.

Robert E. Johnson, PhD, is a biostatistician at Virginia Commonwealth University who holds joint appointments in the Departments of Biostatistics and Family Medicine and is director of data services for the Virginia Commonwealth University Center on Human Needs.

Renate G. Justin, MD, is a retired family physician. She continues to write and has published in both professional and lay journals.

Steven H. Landers, MD, MPH, is a family doctor and geriatrician at Cleveland Clinic.

David Loxterkamp, MD, is a family physician, writer, runner, and potato farmer who has lived for 3 decades with his family on the coast of Maine.

Jon O. Neher, MD, is a clinical professor of Family Medicine at the University of

Washington (Seattle) and Associate Program Director of Valley Medical Center's Family Medicine Residency (Renton, Washington).

William R. Phillips, MD, MPH, is the Theodore J. Phillips Endowed Professor in Family Medicine at the University of Washington.

Ronald E. Pust, MD, is a general practitioner, grandfather, and observer/teacher of clinical "global health" based at the University of Arizona in Tucson.

Darius A. Rastegar, MD, is a general internist at the Johns Hopkins Bayview Medical Center in Baltimore, Maryland.

Rachel Naomi Remen, MD, is Clinical Professor of Family and Community Medicine at the UCSF School of Medicine where she developed the Healer's Art curriculum, presently taught in more than half of US medical schools and seven countries abroad. She is a medical reformer and pioneer in relationship-centered care whose books, *Kitchen Table Wisdom* and *My Grandfather's Blessings*, have been published in 22 languages.

Marino Rivera is a semiretired businessman working in a community health center doing planning and development for the facility center.

Roger A. Rosenblatt, MD, MPH, MFR, is Professor and Vice Chair of the Department of Family Medicine at the University of Washington School of Medicine in Seattle.

George W. Saba, PhD, is an Associate Director, and Director of Behavioral Sciences of University of California, San Francisco–San Francisco General Hospital Family and Community Medicine Residency Program.

Peter A. de Schweinitz, MD, MSPH, works in family medicine and public health for Tanana Chiefs Conference (Fairbanks, Alaska) and the University of Utah.

John G. Scott, MD, PhD, is a family physician in East Burke, Vermont, and was a 2004 recipient of a Robert Wood Johnson Generalist Physician Faculty Scholar award to study healing relationships between clinicians and patients.

Peter A. Selwyn, MD, MSPH, is Chairman of the Department of Family and Social Medicine at Albert Einstein College of Medicine and author of the memoir *Surviving the Fall: The Personal Journey of an AIDS Doctor*.

Sara G. Shields, MD, MS, is a family physician at the Family Health Center of Worcester, a Clinical Associate Professor of Family Medicine and Community Health at the University of Massachusetts, and coeditor of *Woman-Centered Care in Pregnancy and Childbirth* (Radcliffe, 2010).

Andrew L. Sussman, PhD, MCRP, is a medical anthropologist and Associate Director of RIOS Net, a practice-based research network in the Department of Family and Community Medicine at the University of New Mexico.

Contributors

Paul Thomas, FRCGP, MD, is a general practitioner in West London and Clinical Lead for Ealing Clinical Commissioning Group.

Janet M. Townsend, MD, is a family physician who moved from the Bronx to rural northeastern Pennsylvania to help build a new medical school.

William Ventres, MD, MA, is a US family physician living and teaching in Central America. He is affiliated with both the Oregon Health and Science University and the University of El Salvador.

Teresa J. Villela, MD, is Director of the University of California, San Francisco–San Francisco General Hospital Family and Community Medicine Residency Program.

Steven H. Woolf, MD, MPH, is a professor of family medicine at Virginia Commonwealth University, where he directs the Virginia Commonwealth University Center on Human Needs.

Acknowledgments

My heartfelt thanks to Elizabeth Anderson, Laura McLellan, William L. Miller, and William R. Phillips, for their thoughtful suggestions and important technical support; to Jane Richmond, whose careful reading set a clear and concise tone; to Catherine Watson, writer and teacher extraordinaire, who provided invaluable guidance at just the right moment; to Sandy Broyard, for permission to use the insightful words of Anatole Broyard; and to Keri Anderson, whose inspired poem gave this book its title and framework.

I am forever grateful to Kurt Stange, mentor and friend, who "dwell[s] in Possibility."[1] Your optimism made this book a reality; your support helped it to sing.

During the past decade, many courageous writers have allowed the *Annals of Family Medicine* to consider their reflections. I thank each of them for the privilege.

Reference

1. Johnson TH, editor. *The Complete Poems of Emily Dickinson*. New York, NY: Little, Brown; 1961. p. 327.

This book is dedicated to the memory of Carol Bly and her unwavering passion for a clear and honest voice.

Introduction

The Wonder and the Mystery: 10 Years of Reflections from the Annals of Family Medicine is a remarkable gathering of voices from the front lines of primary care. Speaking honestly, arguing passionately, and singing from the heart, these voices reflect on the power of healing, the many meanings of patient care, and the search for wholeness in health, health care, and life.

The articles in this book were first published in the *Annals of Family Medicine*, a journal dedicated to understanding and improving health and primary care. Each article in this anthology makes a unique contribution to that goal. Some do so through innovative ideas that persuade and challenge; with topics as diverse as global environmental change and jazz music, they expand our vision of what health and health care can and should be. Others further our understanding through the power of story. Personal stories offer "an understanding that cannot be arrived at by any other means,"[1] and this book is brimming with them: unforgettable, real-life stories that capture the intricacies of health care and the humanity at its core.

The subject of this book is the vibrant, unpredictable place where primary care and life intersect. It is territory framed by science, built on relationships, and sustained in communities. Here, primary care becomes more than the practice of medicine. It becomes a human endeavor, with all the perils and possibilities that entails. The book provides a rare opportunity to step inside primary care practice, to delight in the satisfaction and grapple with the uncertainty of caring for people's lives. It allows us to witness the past and present – perhaps even the future – of primary care, in all its fullness.

For all of the insights they provide, the articles in this book offer no easy answers. There are many shades of gray in these reflections. This, it turns out, is one of the most intriguing aspects of the anthology. It is not a tribute to a simple vision of heroic physicians and grateful patients. Instead, it honors our imperfect, heartfelt attempts to come together – physician and patient, old and young, optimist and pessimist – to create wholeness, healing, and health. At a time when medical visits are short and frustration with health care is high, those who value primary care continue to strive for something better: a form of care that "seeks connection" and "integrat[es] parts – pieces of information and teams of people – into a meaningful whole."[2] This collection celebrates that striving.

The phrase, "The Wonder and the Mystery," is borrowed from poet Keri Anderson. Her tribute to a family physician who embraced wonder and mystery (*see* A Public Celebration of a Personal Doctor, by William Phillips and Larry Green, p. 167) captures the book's spirit of awareness and possibility. It is perhaps not surprising that an anthology of reflections from primary care contains an element of mystery; dealing with the unknown and uncertain is one of the hallmarks of primary care practice and a recurring theme in these articles. As for wonder, that "mixture of surprise, curiosity, and sometimes awe,"[3] it is present in each passionate belief, courageous reflection, and remarkable relationship that unfolds here.

One of the wonders of this book is the powerful connection that exists between articles. Although they were published separately over a 10-year period, there is a synchronous quality to the stories and ideas. In some cases they complement one another, adding subtlety and depth to what we know of health and life. In other cases they contrast, reminding us of "the complexity, storminess, and wealth of ... lived experiences."[4] Together, these disparate puzzle pieces create a picture of how health and illness shape our lives and how life shapes primary care. From this cohesive whole – this rich stew of insight and inspiration – common themes emerge: the search for meaning in life's transitions, the profound lessons inherent in caring for one another, and the healing power of simply being present. The book is organized around the following seven themes.

1. *Primary Care at Work*: the daily practice of primary care is intricate and ever-changing. As life's work, it can be joyful, painful, and fulfilling.
2. *Patient Care and Caring*: patient care means caring for one another, and ourselves, with compassion.
3. *Wounds and Healing*: life offers illness, pain, and opportunities to heal.
4. *Connections*: at its core, primary care is about relationships.
5. *Knowledge*: study, experience, and reflection are extraordinary teachers.
6. *The Essence of Family Medicine*: essential attributes of family medicine are key to the future of compassionate care.
7. *Medicine, Society, The World*: context matters in medicine and in life.

In the end, the stories and ideas in *The Wonder and the Mystery: 10 Years of Reflections from the* Annals of Family Medicine are wise and generous guides. With open hearts, they share the search for healing and the grace of discovery.

With resonant and lyrical voices, they remind us that wonder and mystery make life richer and that the soul of primary care endures.

References

1. Greenhalgh T, Hurwitz B. Narrative based medicine: why study narrative? *BMJ*. 1999; 318(7175): 48–50.
2. Stange KC. The generalist approach. *Ann Fam Med.* 2009; 7(3): 198–203.
3. Collins. *Wonder*. www.collinsdictionary.com/dictionary/english/wonder (accessed May 12, 2012).
4. Crabtree BF, Miller WL, editors. *Doing Qualitative Research,* 2nd ed. Thousand Oaks, CA: Sage; 1999. p. xi.

Section 1

Primary Care at Work

If you've ever questioned the complexity of primary care, consider this. Primary care is so inclusive in scope that "all aspects of human existence are legitimate concerns."[1] Patients visit primary care physicians with undefined medical issues – mysteries to be solved – and unspoken concerns. When the unexpected arises, as it often does, the work of primary care clinicians becomes a creative act; like jazz musicians, "they make sense of it and improvise."[2]

In this section, we get a close-up view of the pleasures and challenges of caring for a wide spectrum of people and a broad range of conditions, and we consider the legacy of family medicine as life's work. These articles shine a light on primary care practice, offering us the exceptional opportunity to do the following.

- *Meet Magdalena*, a patient who seems to defy cure, despite physician Peter de Schweinitz's best efforts. Over time, she teaches her doctor that healing is sometimes found where you least expect it.
- *Listen*, as Janet Townsend elicits her patients' concerns. Townsend encourages clinicians to be present to their patients' fears, even within the time constraints of the primary care visit.
- *Experience the intricate thought processes of primary care*: Howard Brody offers the rare opportunity to witness a veteran family physician as he assesses, revises, prioritizes, communicates, follows up – and then does it all again.
- *Dance* with William Ventres – for Ventres, the processes of family medicine are pure joy. He finds rejuvenation not only in addressing medical concerns but also in the give and take – the dance – that is inherent in a profession built on human connection.

- *Search for balance*: Joseph Carrese and Michel Ibrahim reflect, with remarkable honesty, on the personal trade-offs that a career in medicine can entail.
- *Consider ethics and practicality in health care*: Howard Brody asks whether physicians should interact with pharmaceutical sales representatives and makes a case based on moral and pragmatic aspects of medical practice.
- *Contemplate legacies*: family physician David Loxterkamp re-visions the meaning of a life devoted to patient care, as his sense of vocation is replaced by something more humble but no less meaningful.

References

1. Heath I. *The Mystery of General Practice*. London: Nuffield Trust; 1995. p. 26.
2. Miller WL, McDaniel RR Jr, Crabtree BF, et al. Practice jazz: understanding variation in family practices using complexity science. *J Fam Pract*. 2001; 50(10): 872–78.

1

Nasruddin and the Coin

Peter A. de Schweinitz, MD, MSPH

WHEN I WAS A BOY, MY DAD, AN ELECTRICAL ENGINEER OF SOLID European stock, told me Middle Eastern stories, most often about Nasruddin, a wise fool and wanderer. One dark night Nasruddin arrived in a village to find a man searching about under a street lamp. He approached the man and asked what he was looking for. "A gold coin," came the reply. After searching with the man for a few minutes, Nasruddin asked the man where he had lost it.

The man pointed across the street. "Over there," he said.

"Well why are we looking for it here?" Nasruddin replied.

The man looked at Nasruddin in disbelief. "There's no light over there."

Many problems can be understood and treated by the light of diagnostic and therapeutic algorithms and common biomedical knowledge. There are other problems and situations in which rubrics, biochemical markers, images, consultants, and medicines fail to help the patient. As physicians, what do we do with our patients when the answers are not forthcoming? At times, both physician and patient must crawl around in the dark.

During the autumn of my family medicine internship, a 38-year-old Latina transferred care from the community health center to my clinic. A social wallflower with a bowl-cut hairdo, white tennis shoes, and unshapely slacks, Magdalena looked to me with a respect I'd hardly yet earned. "I have insurance now," she explained, "so I can come to a better clinic." I felt a twinge of guilt; her former physicians were some of my best teachers.

Born with a "bad kidney," Magdalena had been diagnosed in her Caribbean homeland with hypertension when she was just 13 years old. Ten years later, after immigrating with her family to Florida, her bad kidney was identified and removed. Sometime in the interim she met missionaries and left Catholicism for a Protestant denomination, then moved westward to the Rocky Mountains to be close to fellow believers. While studying family science at the local university, she suffered a cerebrovascular accident. The stroke did not take her ability to reason and speak, but did leave her with mild weakness and a slight limp. She now lived alone and depressed, in a small apartment just outside of the university campus.

For the next two and one-half years I tried to help Magdalena. First, there was her recalcitrant blood pressure. I spent the initial six months ruling out secondary causes of hypertension and searching for the ideal medical regimen. I examined her single remaining renal artery with magnetic resonance imaging and checked her urine catecholamine levels. I titrated her medications, and I added and switched classes of medicine. Despite my best efforts (and the guidance of the faculty physicians), by her sixth visit to the clinic, her blood pressure had decreased only slightly, from 156/95 mm Hg to 148/90 mm Hg.

For her depression, I tried paroxetine, sertraline, and venlafaxine. At times Magdalena seemed encouraged, imagining that she was healed. But her improvements never lasted. Most likely the medicines never rendered an effect beyond the temporary placebo response, which seemed to correlate with Magdalena's hopeful and pleasing attitude toward her inexperienced doctor.

By the spring of my intern year I had neither succeeded in reducing her blood pressure nor in alleviating her depression. Moreover, she suffered a first seizure. An attending physician blamed the seizure on her prior stroke. I suspected my failure to control her blood pressure was more likely responsible. Magdalena, however, heaped blame on herself, on her fate. "Yo suffro mucho [I suffer much]," she said.

"Maybe she should see a counselor," I said.

Our faculty behavioral medicine director didn't see the point. George rocked back in his chair, elevating his Green Bay Packers tie to the brim of his ample paunch. "What is it that she would talk to them about?"

"I don't know. Maybe they could help her to see things differently."

But George must have lost faith in psychotherapy as a magic bullet. "Does she *want* to see a counselor?"

"No, I don't think so," I said.

"What I like to do is start with the primary arenas," he said. "Work, religion, and family."

The next few months were filled with strenuous encounters. As I broadened the scope of our interviews, I learned about Magdalena's father, the diligent electrician; her mother, the loyal homemaker; and of Magdalena's devotion to her new religious community. At times Magdalena's eyes welled with tears, especially when talking of her parents, both now dead. Often catharsis seemed to bring Magdalena peace, but in the end this seeming peace would quickly fade, as had any benefit of the antidepressants. I wondered whether self-discovery and emotional expression were of any permanent value.

"How do we change people, George?"

George's tie inched a button or so up his green sweater. "I figure we give 'em what we have, and they take what they want. We know we're done when they stop showing up."

Although in general I admired George, I couldn't quickly absorb his wisdom. To my young mind, his shotgun approach seemed overly passive (even blasé). As a professional, wasn't I supposed to precisely diagnose and choose from my doctor's bag the one best remedy for the circumstance? George made medicine sound like a Sunday morning buffet.

Despite my skepticism, I attempted to incorporate the advice of my mentor by opening up a separate and more personal bag of remedies, those which had worked in my own life. Thich Nhat Hanh had written about "mindful" walking; I skipped the Buddhist references and simply suggested a walk to clear the head. At church I'd learned that prayer can release emotional tension and yield divine guidance; I made the suggestion. (We shared a religion.) Viktor Frankl and Rachel Remen had written of the therapeutic importance of discovering life's meaning; I suggested journaling. Sometimes George's advice seemed to make sense. Magdalena walked out with hope. She always returned, however, with the same limp and the same pleasing smile that would ultimately give way to her downturned gaze and slumped shoulders.

With time I learned more about Magdalena and her loneliness. A single woman in a familial community, Magdalena saw marriage as an essential element of existence, mandatory, in fact, for both true happiness and "eternal progression." Around her, students one-half her age were dating, proposing, and projecting themselves into the future through their offspring. Magdalena's parents had long since died, and her fertile years were coming to a close.

"Do you ever go out, Magdalena?"

"Claro que si [Yes, of course], Doctor. I go to church parties sometimes." Magdalena answered my hesitant question with a superficial answer. "On Friday we played a game of Frisbee at the park." At the time I couldn't imagine Magdalena attracting a mate. I looked at her and saw a stroke victim and spinster, a soul with little hope of happiness, in terms both American culture and her religion prescribed.

Then, two months before I graduated from residency, something unusual happened: Magdalena missed her monthly appointment. By this point, Magdalena had begun to blend into the crowd of chronic patients – the type who trigger the smile of habit, the professional nod, and the rote medication renewal. Thoughts of her no longer pestered me on the bike ride home from the clinic or entered dinner conversations with my wife and young son. In short, I had lost hope (nearly) for a cure. And George's philosophy – "give 'em what we have and they take what they want" – seemed less blasé and more realistic, perhaps even wise, if only as a method of lowering one's expectations.

It was only after my medical assistant handed me her chart that I realized that I hadn't seen Magdalena in two months. I looked at the yellow sticky note on her chart. Then I looked again. I practically scowled at my assistant. "Are these right?" Her blood pressure was 125/82 mm Hg! The young woman nodded. Frowning not so much at the assistant as at this deviation from the expected – this normal pressure in a recalcitrant hypertensive – I opened the door.

I've only twice in my medical career seen a patient so abruptly changed – once when I halved the dose of long-acting methylphenidate on a 10-year-old-turned-zombie, and the other time when a smoker gave up cigarettes and began to oxygenate.

Magdalena had never been assertive, but now she came after me like an old pal. "How have you been, Doctor?" I sat down on my stool. "The weather has been so nice these days, you know, not too hot."

I cut in: "Where have you been, Magdalena?"

"Florida." For the first time in many years Magdalena had visited her only remaining close family member, an aunt.

"Look at that," I said, pointing at the sticky note.

Magdalena smiled. "I know, Doctor. I had to stop one of my medicines. I was getting dizzy."

"Dizzy, like the room was spinning, or light headed, like you were going to faint?"

"Light headed," she replied.

"What happened?"

Magdalena recounted her visit to the Florida hospital, where the emergency department doctor had ordered her to stop one of her two blood pressure medicines. Magdalena was not intrigued with her sudden drop in blood pressure, but I was. Even success – a patient's improvement – is not enough. We need an explanation. "Is that all you did in Florida, Magdalena ... see your aunt?"

Magdalena's eyes flicked low and oblique. She paused briefly, as if allowing any distracting inhibition to pass. "While I was there, I saw a man I used to know."

Drawing on my images of Florida – a state I'd never visited – and on our many conversations about her early family experiences, I imagined her at a dingy apartment complex, speaking with an elderly friend of her deceased father. Dusty toys littered the floor of the stairwell.

"What did you talk about, Magdalena?"

Magdalena's eyes dropped once again to the floor. This time they returned solemn with authority. "Doctor, 20 years ago I was engaged to be married." With one sentence my image of Magdalena had shattered. Wasn't she a 41-year-old spinster with a limp? For the first time I recognized the attractive radiance of her dark brown eyes.

"In the winter you told me to write in my journal. You remember?"

I didn't. "Oh, yeah. Uh huh."

"I wrote in my journal, Doctor. Every day, like you said. I hadn't even remembered him until I started writing. When I was in Florida I decided to go find him. I looked him up in the telephone book. I asked him why he did that to me, why he broke off the engagement. You know what he told me, Doctor?" I shook my head. "He said it wasn't about me. He said it was because of his own problems. All this time I thought I was too ugly or not good enough."

For 20 years Magdalena had lived with an assumption. That assumption had lived in her hesitant smile and formless clothing. It reflected back at her through the words, actions, and subtle gestures of her social world. Even her doctor, someone who had wanted badly to make her world better, could not see her differently. Perhaps for a time Magdalena tried to wear a smile over her assumption. She covered it over with a new life out West, with Frisbee in the park, with a new apartment or new part-time job. Then somehow she forgot it altogether. But it did not forget her. A fragment of Magdalena's life remained where she had dropped it.

Like the men in the old tale, Magdalena and I began our relationship by searching for the coin under the safety of the street lamp by using the standard algorithms of care. Sometimes, however, what lies at the root of uncontrolled disease is outside the obvious medical causes. Unique and personal factors may underlie, anchor, or interact with the patient's chronic problem or behavior. (This may be true even when the antihypertensive drug works.) What do we do when the textbook fails to heal the patient? Do we continue to invite the patient back month after month? When she comes, how do we spend our time? Sometimes we must leave the easy certainty of the lamp. We trip across the road, get down on our hands and knees, and search.

2

One Last Question

Opening Pandora's Box?

Janet M. Townsend, MD

IT HAD BEEN A TYPICAL MONDAY MORNING AT THE TEACHING PRACTICE where I see patients, though patient flow was chaotic as we implemented a new registration system. I was running a few patients behind and regretting that my patients had to wait so long. Mrs B was next. I had assumed her care several months before. A 70-year-old retired licensed practical nurse with diabetes, hypertension, and recent leg edema, Mrs B always seemed well-informed and on top of things.

This time I was concerned because her serum creatinine had risen far above her baseline. I informed her, and she seemed surprised that there would be any problem with her kidneys, even though her creatinine had hovered around 1.3 mg/dL for several years. Her previous physician had ordered a renal sonogram last year, which she had understood to be normal. We discussed, in a matter-of-fact way, the possible causes of the decline in kidney function and decided to repeat the laboratory tests and a urinalysis. We also anticipated what would be involved in further work-up if the laboratory results confirmed the change in her creatinine level.

I shuffled papers in the chart to review any previous evaluation and her medication list, struggled with a new laboratory requisition sheet, and checked on her routine monitoring for diabetes and last mammogram. I was already past the 15 minutes allotted for her visit. Mrs B answered all my questions clearly and confidently. Just as I was about to hand Mrs B the laboratory orders and appointment slip and pick up the chart to leave, I stopped, put everything down, and looked her in the eye.

"Mrs B, I rushed so much to take care of everything today – we talked about the kidney problem rather quickly. How are you feeling about all this?"

"Scared to death, Doctor, scared to *death*," she said, without blinking an eye. "Everyone in my family has kidney trouble – my mother, my uncle. I have two sisters on dialysis." Her eyes filled with tears.

"Then you've been dreading this?" I asked.

What was it that made me pause to ask that key question about how she was feeling? I had been close to walking out the door without grasping how worried she was. Yet I did pause, for those few seconds of silence, to look once more at the patient, to connect. We took a few more minutes to talk about her fears. I assured her that I would let her know the results promptly, and that I anticipated an early consultation with a nephrologist. She left the office looking somewhat relieved, expecting to wait several days for the results.

Later that week, I returned to the office for some patient follow-up and chart review. One of our medical assistants asked me to handle an authorization and referral for a vacationing colleague. It was for an ultrasound-guided breast biopsy for a patient whose mammogram revealed a lesion. The patient was a 68-year-old woman in good health who I didn't know. Not wanting to write the referral without checking with the patient, I called her at home and had the following conversation.

"Hello, Mrs M, this is Dr Townsend. I work with Dr P, who is on vacation. I understand you had to go back to the hospital to get some other x-rays of your breast."

"Yes, Doctor," she said, a Caribbean lilt in her voice.

"Did they tell you they had seen a spot, a lump that needs a biopsy?"

"Yes, Doctor."

"Did they schedule the biopsy?"

"Yes, Doctor, next Tuesday."

"Is that OK with you? Do you understand what they are going to do?

"Yes, Doctor."

"And you'll be able to go?"

"Yes, Doctor."

"I'll write the referral for Dr P and everything will be set."

"Yes, Doctor."

"And I'll tell Dr P when he gets back."

"Yes, Doctor."

After a brief silence, I was about to say good-bye when I asked one more question, perhaps in hopes of getting an answer beyond the deferential, "Yes, Doctor."

"Mrs M, are you worried about this?"

"Oh, yes, Doctor," a near-sob in her voice.

"You're worried you have cancer?"

"Yes, Doctor."

"Have you told anyone about this?

"No, Doctor."

We talked for a few more minutes, about how mammograms help us find cancers early and whether she could talk to a family member or friend about her worries. She promised to talk about it with her daughter, and I promised to call the radiologist to learn more about what they saw on her mammogram. I urged her not to worry alone. Later on that day, I called Mrs M to let her know that the radiologist said the lesion was very small.

In our busy practice lives, we can easily miss the worry beneath the surface of our conversations with patients. As a family doctor, confident of my skills in integrating inquiry about psychosocial issues in routine care and committed to training young physicians in this model, I was surprised that I had come close to ignoring this key dimension in these two encounters. Had I been misled by the competence of Mrs B or the reserve of Mrs M? Had my use of closed-ended questions, seemingly appropriate for a simple telephone call or for discussing laboratory results, limited what the patients could tell me? Was I distracted by the confusion and delays in the practice that first day, or was I simply hurrying because I was running behind? Did my intention to make a brief stop at the practice to do "just a few things" limit my openness to clues from Mrs M?

Yet I did pause to ask the one last question, the one that allowed these patients to reveal their worry. A psychologist colleague always reminds us that including just one question on the psychosocial dimension in every visit is likely to pay off. I've found her advice to be true over the years. Even when hurried and hassled, the visit feels incomplete without making room for that final check-in with the patient about the meaning or impact of what we've said. Silence, pauses, eye contact, a last question – these ingrained habits serve as a check on a premature end to the visit and assure a connection with the patient.

We often worry that such questions will open Pandora's box, the one opened by that much-maligned goddess who, in Greek mythology, unleashed all the ills of the world. Truly, we physicians are messengers of Pandora's problem-filled world. We connect patients to that world, almost as immediately as aches and pains do. In a way it is our job to open Pandora's box – we question, we probe, we order tests, we name risks, we raise issues patients would just as soon leave alone. We play Pandora. We connect patients to their illness. We can't avoid it. It's what we do.

Yet our curiosity and our questions can lead to insights into the patient's world that help us to share worry and isolation or to mobilize support from family and friends. In this regard, it is interesting to recall that after Pandora opened her box, letting loose all that chaos, she managed to shut it just in time to prevent hope from escaping. As physicians, by connecting to patients through simple personal questions, we connect them to hope. In small ways, our attention to patients' unspoken fears helps to maintain that emotional quality, hope, so essential to well-being. And hope springs not only from positive prognoses and reassurance that we may be able to offer, but also from the power of patients' own reflections, their ability to name fears and to solve problems, and their willingness to ask for help from others. In Greek, after all, Pandora means "all gifts." We, too, are endowed with gifts as a result of our training, the diagnostic tools and treatment options at our disposal, an ever-expanding medical and scientific knowledge, and the wisdom gained through experience, which we offer to patients. By opening Pandora's box, we make room for listening, for reflection, and for putting things into perspective, and with our gifts, we open doors for healing.

We should embrace Pandora's curiosity and her courage. Perhaps we need not fear opening Pandora's box, but rather we should fear leaving it shut.

I want to offer a final note, having just returned from a gathering of the leaders of our discipline at the Association of Departments of Family Medicine winter meeting. I believe this moment is precious and unique in medicine, when mounting evidence documents the value of family medicine and primary care in keeping people healthy and in reducing mortality. We will have many new tools at our fingertips in the coming decades, including medications tailored to individual genetic patterns, ever more amazing imaging techniques, and less-invasive approaches to surgery. Yet, the processes of care upon which family medicine is built and the relationships that ensue may be our most powerful tool of all. As my new Dean notes, "Listening is the cornerstone of medicine."

Let us raise our collective voice in support of a system of care that makes room for listening – to patients, to each other, and to communities.

3

A Headache at the End of the Day

Howard Brody, MD, PhD

GLANCE DOWN AT THE BOTTOM OF THE SCHEDULE TO SEE WHO'S THE last patient. Larry Wong, headache. Not one of my regular patients; a sick call. Hope it's quick. Tonight I have to meet my wife for dinner. For some crazy reason, I am nearly on time finishing up with my next-to-last patient. I see the encounter form on the door of the other examination room, but the room is empty. "Your last patient isn't here yet," says the aide. "His father checked him in, but he's coming with his mother, and they're not here yet."

Father? Mother? I figured it must be an adult, coming in with a headache. Nope – here it is, 5 years old. Not too many 5-year-olds complain of headache. Wonder what's going on. Both parents coming, too? A big deal. At least their being late is no problem; I can work on my notes for other patients.

Okay, he's finally here. Encounter form says they usually see Dr Price. Say hello – great, the parents speak good English. Shake hands with Larry. First agenda: establish rapport, I am going to treat him like an adult, I'll take him seriously. Next agenda: support the relationship with the primary doc, don't get into competition with my partner. "I'm sorry that Dr Price must have had a full schedule today; I'll try to fill in as best as I can till you can see him."

So now, what's the problem? I look at Larry, but it's unlikely a 5-year-old will start talking with both parents in the room. Sure enough, Dad takes over. A 2-day history of complaints of frontal headache, swollen and red left eyelid, feeling tired, no fever. Took him to the lake yesterday, Sunday, but he said he felt tired and sick, and kept putting his hands in front of his eyes as if the light hurt. This morning, got up, the swelling was gone. Now he says he feels fine, they report.

Mom is holding tight to his two medicines – a corticosteroid inhaler and a bottle of nonsedating antihistamine tablets. They didn't give him the tablets this morning, she says, they were worried the tablets might be causing his headache. Hmm. The antihistamine may be pricey, but it hardly ever causes headaches that I've heard. Why would they think it was the culprit?

Glance at the computer screen while they are talking. Problem list: mild intermittent asthma, allergic rhinitis, history of pneumonia. No clear reason why they'd be bringing a child in to the doctor when his problems had gotten better on their own. A lot of visits recently for a pretty healthy kid, too. Mom seems worried. She throws in something about him not eating right.

Next agenda: the differential. Nothing is coming to mind that's serious and that would cause a headache like this that seems to have gone away on its own. Light hurts – photophobia. Migraine? Unlikely at this age.

Dad is still talking, and now Larry starts to say something. I've got to keep my promise to Larry to take him seriously, but I want to hear what Dad is going to say. I am still trying to get a handle on what the parents are worried about. Look Larry in the eye: "Larry, I need to let your Dad finish, and then it will be your turn." He looks me back in the eye. Great, he buys it.

Now Dad's finished. "Okay, Larry, now it's your turn." Showing him I'll keep my promises at least. Larry is a typical 5-year-old, runs to Dad to whisper in his ear, won't tell me directly. Uh oh, trouble – Dad is telling Larry he should talk to me, not be afraid. Worried his kid is embarrassing the family in front of the doctor. Touchy. I have to give Larry breathing room but not seem to be undermining Dad's authority. Give it a shot: "Dad, I want to ask you for a big favor. It's real normal for 5-year-olds to be pretty shy in the office here – it's not their usual environment." Try to normalize the behavior – nothing to feel ashamed of. "So maybe you could let him whisper to you and then tell me." Relief: Dad is taking it all right, he does not look upset. Larry whispers to Dad and Dad starts to tell me, and as I expect, Larry breaks in and tells me anyway. No biggie, just wants to change the order in which he had the symptoms – says he felt tired first and then had the headache later. "Do you feel okay now?" The parents already told me that, but now we have Larry's role in the conversation established, so that's good.

Next agenda: I'm an unknown, not their usual doctor. They are worried. Gotta' do a pretty thorough physical or they won't be satisfied. Also on the agenda: standard 5-year-old stuff, get the kid to cooperate and have fun with the examination.

Head is normal, I don't see any redness or swelling of the eyelids. Neck is supple. Pupils equal and reactive to light, discs look fine. Larry's cooperating nicely as I would have expected. "How wide can you open your mouth?" Plenty wide, no need for a tongue depressor. "When Dr Price looks in your ears, does he look for anything special? Frogs? Butterflies? Potatoes?" Larry looks from me to his Dad – why are you letting this lunatic examine me? "Well, okay, we'll just look in and see what we see." He holds still just fine. "You're right – no frogs or butterflies." Ears are clear bilaterally. Throat is normal. Neck has no nodes.

"Take big breaths in and out like this." No wheezes. "Great – he sounds fine" – to Mom. "Do you know where your heart is?" Larry points. "Great – let's listen. I'll listen first and then you can." I take the ear pieces out of my ears and hand them over to Larry while holding the diaphragm in place. Dad is now into it and helps Larry put the ear pieces in his ears. Larry grins as he hears the heartbeat. Okay, just about done, abdominal examination and we have probably done enough to make the parents happy. Everything normal. Still no clue as to what the real worries are. Gotta' get to that next – maybe now the parents will trust me enough to say what's on their minds.

"Just as you suspected" – let's make it partly their idea – "Larry checks out just fine now. Plus his asthma seems to be under good control with the medicines." Now Dad pipes up, wants to know more about the asthma. Oh – he was away in China when they made the diagnosis, this is his first visit to the office since Larry was labeled an asthmatic. Bingo. Goes off to China and his kid is fine, all of a sudden his kid is sick, running back and forth to the office, has a major illness label stuck on him. No wonder he's worried. It's starting to make some sense. Thank goodness they're the last patients of the day; I've got time.

How to get Dad to feel back in the loop? Well, computers always know the answers, right? Time for the electronic record to strut its stuff. "Here, let's pull up to the computer screen and we'll look at the recent office visits one at a time and figure out just what happened in order." Stupid me, too busy getting my other charts done, didn't bother to read the previous notes before going in the room. Figured it was just a routine sick call and I could wing it. Gotta' get back on track. "Well, first thing we see is that Dr Price has called it mild intermittent asthma. That's the least serious kind." See if that helps. Yes, he looks relieved. "It looks here like they did some lab tests" – elevated IgE – "plus Larry seemed to have a cough that held on for a long time after he had a cold, often that's the first sign of a mild asthma. Now here, he came in to see Dr Burns for a sick call, he tried an albuterol inhaler, and the cough got a lot better, it says." Mom nods. "So that also goes along with a mild asthma."

So why did they jump right in with an inhaled corticosteroid? "Here's the next note, back with Dr Price. It says that Larry was going to go to China too, and they were worried about the air pollution making the asthma worse, so he decided at least for a while to use the daily medicine. Larry, did you go to China?" No, says Mom, we were too worried about him getting sick; right after his diagnosis of asthma, he came down with a cold, so we canceled the trip. Whoa – major big-time anxiety here. Probably whatever is at the bottom of this is a lot more than I can handle in one sick call visit. Now I understand what Dad is worried about. He was planning to see his wife and kid, having them join him in China; all of a sudden the kid is too sick to come, he's halfway around the world and can't do anything. No wonder he freaked. Is his wife upset with him, putting his career first and leaving her with all the child care responsibility? Forgot to ask what work he does; he looks like a university professor type, which is typical for our practice. Stupid me again – should have asked to be sure. Don't want to change the subject just now, though.

Next agenda: see what I can do by way of reassurance as the nonprimary doc. "I wonder if you folks have had the same experience as a lot of parents that we see. Just by bad luck, a healthy kid has a few illnesses in a row. Then in just a couple of months, he's back to being healthy as usual. But the parents get worried and are afraid that he has something wrong with him, like an immune deficiency or something. But really it's just temporary bad luck." They're nodding, maybe they buy it. "Plus I think it's perfectly okay to go back to using the antihistamine, because this is the allergy season and if he has worse allergies, his asthma might get worse again. I don't think that the antihistamine was the cause of his head-ache." Maybe better back off a little, don't seem to be contradicting them too much. "Of course, if you go back on it and he has another headache, and then his headache gets better if you stop it again, then we'll think differently." That should cover the bases, show I'm keeping an open mind.

Dad now wants to know, if asthma is an immune reaction, and the antihista-mine works for allergies and asthma, won't it suppress his immune system too much, maybe he'll get more colds? Bingo again. Now we know why they were so worried about the antihistamine. Sounds perfectly logical when you think about it – I wonder why no other patient has ever asked me that. Good thing I said the magic words "immune deficiency" – maybe that triggered them asking what was really on their minds. If so, I stumbled into that one by pure dumb luck. "You know, that's a *really* good question. The good news is that the antihistamine is a very targeted drug – it shuts down the one part of the immune system that's directly related to allergic reactions, but it leaves alone all the parts that fight infection." Should I go into mast cells and histamines? No; it looks like he's satisfied.

Okay, back to the primary doc agenda. "Would it be all right if I set up an appointment for all of you to see Dr Price again as soon as he has an opening?

We want him to check up on how Larry's asthma is doing, plus he may want to take him off the steroid inhaler for now, since he didn't end up going to China and won't have to deal with the air pollution. I'll sure write a careful note today to let Dr Price know all that we talked about." That works, they seem fine with that. Now it's the big ceremony of the Sticker Drawer for Larry, and they're out of here.

Did I help out at all, really? First I'm pretty sure that Larry's not sick and the headache is no big deal. Did I do anything to reduce the parental anxiety level? Probably not. I still don't know what's going on in Mom's head. Or for that matter what the real relationship is between Mom and Dad. She may be back in with Larry in three days with another minor complaint. Gotta' remember to ask Price to keep me posted on how these folks do down the road. And better write a more detailed note than usual.

Speaking of writing my notes, what time is it now? My gosh – I spent half an hour with them, when I was supposed to be getting out of here on time. Now, just why did I spend that extra time? I thought that the parents needed to be reassured, plus I had to be sure we included Larry in the visit, too. These things take time; you can't always rush good family medicine.

Then it hit me. The other reason why I took the extra time: I was enjoying myself. In fact, I was having a ball in there.

4

The Joy of Family Practice

William Ventres, MD, MA

Remember the book The Joy of Sex? *I would like to write a book,* The Joy of Family Practice. *There is a tremendous amount of gratification and satisfaction that can come from this kind of medical practice. We as physicians have the opportunity to develop the doctor-patient relationship to an incredible degree.*

It's really an incredibly fulfilling undertaking, and it makes it worthwhile to get up in the middle of the night to go out and see somebody or to spend the time necessary and do whatever you can to help people.

It gets back to the family – it's a way of becoming part of that person's family. That, to me, is more important than the salary, the benefits, and the prestige of being a doctor, and I think it's much more sustaining.

—Lynn Carmichael[1]

Introduction

Two decades ago I had the privilege of interviewing Lynn Carmichael, one of the early leaders of the modern family medicine movement and the founder of the Society of Teachers of Family Medicine. I was new to practice, fresh out of a family medicine residency and a research fellowship. Lynn was one among many elder statesmen in the discipline. I didn't yet know what it meant to be a family physician – it took me quite some time in community practice to figure it out – and Lynn seemed so eloquent in his deep knowledge and understanding.

For years I hoped to read Lynn's book, the one to which he alluded in our interview: "The Joy of Family Practice." But it never got written. Lynn had other responsibilities, I am sure, as chair of the Department of Family Medicine and Community Health at the University of Miami. Later he was afflicted with Alzheimer's disease and slowly, over years, lost his exuberance, his creativity, and his presence. All but a shadow of the Lynn I interviewed was gone. Then in 2009 he died.[2]

I have hoped, too, that in the absence of Lynn's ability to write of his joy in practice, someone else would write explicitly about the personal joy of being a family physician. To be sure, there are many who have touched on the subject. Our colleagues Lucy Candib,[3] David Loxterkamp,[4] John Frey,[5] and many others in the United States have spoken to issues of relationship and community as family physicians. So have practitioners from other parts of the world, including Canada,[6] the United Kingdom,[7] the Iberian Peninsula,[8] and Latin America,[9,10] where family medicine of one variant or another forms the foundation of their respective health care systems. Still, I have wanted to read of what the work of family medicine brings to us as professionals, as individuals, as people.

So rather than wait another 20 years, and with the understanding that I enter into the written expression of my joys as an exploration rather than as a pronouncement, here I write my "Joy of Family Practice." It is not a book – as a doctor in practice I have become accustomed to beginning and finishing tasks in short blocks of time. It is not a universal truth – what I write is born of my particular training and practice and my own signature responses. It is not complete – at 54 years of age I anticipate many years of practice ahead of me.

This "Joy of Family Practice," however, is my joy. It is a brief summary of why I keep coming back, day to day, month to month, year to year, and moment to moment, to do the work I do. It is a love story of sorts, an expression of my appreciation for the work I have chosen as a family physician – rich, engaging, and fulfilling – and, as such, it is with love I begin.

Love

Love is clearly a complex and easily misunderstood word, but I still enjoy using it to describe both what I bring to my practice and what I receive in return from my patients. Many years ago I read the Mexican poet and Nobel Laureate Octavio

Paz's *The Labyrinth of Solitude*, in which he defined love as "a perpetual discovery, an immersion into the waters of reality, and an unending recreation."[11,12] I have yet to find a definition that works better for me as I put into words what I hope I offer to patients in examination rooms or hospital suites. To be sure, it has measures of mindfulness and presence and the Rogerian concept of unconditional positive regard,[13–15] but at its essence the love I speak of is filled with an awe of exploration that permeates my encounters with patients. Who is this person? Who is accompanying him or her? Why are they here? With what issues do they present, and what unsaid concerns lie behind their chief complaints? What are their struggles and where are their resiliencies?

That I am a family physician and not a psychiatrist means that the expression of this love is not solely bound by the world of words, but has physical elements as well. Auscultating heart sounds or palpating an abdomen with compassion, not lacking of sensitivity, does as much to create avenues of communication as does opening my ears to hear my patients' suffering and distress. That I am a family physician and not a subspecialist means that this expression is not bound by barriers of organ system, procedural domain, gender, or age, but is at once inclusive and expansive. It is a love expressed wherever the patient concern might be. That I am a family physician means, too, that this love is expressed with humility. In one sense, it is for the most part focused around everyday matters, both chronic concerns with which people walk the paths of their lives, and acute, generally short-term problems that occasionally show up on those paths as pebbles to be tripped over. In another sense, it is given in recognition that little things take on meanings much larger than they may seem. The welcoming attention I offer may be the single most important thing my patients receive that day – or that year.

In return, I am greeted with a reciprocal sense of love, a respect, a trust, and an invitation to join with my patients as they make their ways in life, with gratitude when things go well as well as when they do not. My patients know that I am not infallible – I do not represent myself as such and am ready to admit my limitations – but they know that I will be there for them as much as is possible in the context of their medical concerns. As a family physician, I am greeted with love born of the understanding that we are more alike than dissimilar, that we are more connected than alone, and that – professional role notwithstanding – we are on a common journey through illness and pain, through difficulty and infirmity as well as joy.

Faith

Family medicine and family practice used to be considered two different sides of the same coin. Family medicine was the academic discipline, the research and teaching. Family practice was what one did in offices and hospitals, the daily work of attending to patients. For marketing and political reasons, more than anything else, "practice" was dropped and the work of family physicians was subsumed under family medicine. Yet I consider my work still a practice. It is a studied practice, one with knowledge and skills and scientific acumen. It is also a practice of faith.

The faith I refer to is not some dogmatic adherence to a set of beliefs or unquestioning surrender to someone else's authority, both of which seem to have created "turf" mentalities that divide people. It is a faith that by being open to patients as people in the context of medical encounters, something more thera-peutic happens than is possible when strictly biomedical necessities are attended to. There exists a shared sense of possibility, a shared potential, and a shared understanding that leads us to go forward even when life is difficult or uncertain. It is a practiced faith in that, as a family physician, I must constantly be aware of looking for that potential, wherever it may exist in context of my patients' lives. It is a practiced faith, too, in that this abiding understanding helps support me in a work that is often challenging and occasionally baffling.

My work is a practice of faith because it draws on a worldview that is interdependent and inexplicable, much more complex than the reductionistic biomedical model that I was taught in medical school and residency. So many factors influence the health of my patients – diseases, behaviors, family dynamics, race, sex, geography, political climate, and money are but some of them. It is my job to sift through these with patients and, with intelligence, discernment, and heart, assist them in seeing the possibilities latent within change and help them move forward. Even when lives are not tidy and manageable or predictable – and they rarely are in the face of illness – I am there to observe, to recognize, to bear witness to, and to offer a path amidst the unknown.

Mystery

Among other reasons, family medicine is challenging because it deals with uncertainty, and I often think that it is my tolerance for uncertainty that sets me apart from my subspecialist colleagues. I deal with uncertainty, first, because my patients present with what are commonly poorly defined, undifferentiated problems, and these problems reflect a variety of possibly related or unrelated causal forces or events. Second, like most family physicians, I generally see patients in short blocks of time. Any sense of increasing certainty rarely comes to me instantaneously but rather over repeated visits with my patients. This sense is enhanced by an awareness of the communities in which my patients live, as well as by our understanding of how my patients live in those communities. Third, because I am a true generalist, there will always be an overabundance of information for me as a family physician to assimilate.

I was trained to look for and see information in objectified bits and pieces as a means to lessen doubt – and I should add that this created within me an oppressive feeling of anxiety – but over time I have come to see uncertainty as something to be accepted as part of my work. It is not as though I have abandoned compulsiveness as a strategy to cope with uncertainty – physicians for the most part share this characteristic to some extent – but I have learned that uncertainty is less to be feared and avoided than to be creatively engaged as a mystery to be explored.[16] It is as though I lean into the vague ambiguities that are inherent in the work I do, expecting there to be stories behind the pain and suffering my patients present with, knowing that I will not hear them all, believing that it is through time and trust and respect and insight – appreciating my own abilities as a family physician to listen in context – that they will become evident, as is needed, as is important, and as is clinically relevant.

Place

The way I conceptualize my work as a family physician probably puts me on the periphery of allopathic medicine, where the hegemony of biomedical thinking reigns. Medical schools overwhelmingly teach their students from a Flexnerian foundation that prioritizes particularized knowledge at the expense of an integrated understanding of disease and health across the biopsychosocial spectrum.[17,18] For the most part even family medicine residencies train their residents in such manners and settings that suggest that family practice is but the compilation of sets of knowledge, mostly modeled after subspecialty practice and mostly taught in hospitals or their associated clinics. Ironically, it has been some community-based subspecialists who have best understood my work. I suspect that while they recognize my limitations of knowledge among the patients I refer to them for consultation, they also recognize their own limitations in understanding the complexities of patient care outside the boundaries of conventional medicine – where my expertise lies.

At one and the same time, I find satisfaction knowing that my work positions me at the core of why so many people entered medicine: to bring care to people; to offer hope when possible and solace when needed; to cure when it is a reasonable goal, to manage and support when it is not. From an organizational perspective, family medicine is an eminently logical foundational layer within a rational health care system, and I am extremely proud to be a very small part of that foundation. But we do not have a rational system of care here in the United States,[19] and it is difficult and often lonely to avoid the strong pulls that money and status and ideology present in our country. As for me, I take refuge in accepting that there are more important things in life than those that can be conferred by the traditional accoutrements of our culture. I also know the central role I play in my patients' lives, as a counselor, as a guide, and as their personal physician.

Dance

It is in my role as personal physician that I sometimes find myself figuratively dancing at work. My fashion sense is not flashy, my moves are not fancy, and I have been known to miss beats and step on toes occasionally. But there is an undeniable elegance to what I am doing, to how I am interacting, and to the knowledge and skills and attitude that I bring to my encounters with patients. I find myself dancing with patients when there is a give and take between us, giving space for each one of us to lead and follow when it is most appropriate. When I lead, my intent is to help my patients and their families to feel a sense of competency in the face of challenge. When I follow, it is to allow them room to express their fears as well as their own special strengths. I find myself dancing with my patients when the rhythm of their needs and my responses create some mutually resonant rapport. I find myself dancing with them when, after the 10 or 15 or 25 minutes of our visit is done and the tasks of problem list review and medication reconciliation and charting are completed and I am leaving the examination room, I can honestly say, "I'll be thinking about you. Until our next visit."

When we are dancing, there is a flow between my patients and me that suggests connections beyond the examination room, residual reverberations of words and movements and intents. There is a temporal connection that extends well after the office visit is over, one that I believe helps direct their welfare at the same time it nurtures my well-being. There is a human connection, too, one that extends to and is amplified by the people around us, the receptionists and nurses and laboratory technicians and social workers with whom I work. As well, there is a spatial connection that helps all our lives become more expansive, more readily willing to grow, and more conscious of kindness to self and others in the face of adversity. The art of the dance is, ultimately, about dignity and grace across dimensions of time and person and place, about sharing a generosity of spirit when the despair of illness threatens, and allowing the effects of that generosity to linger well after my patients and I part.

Medicine

The foundation of what I do as a family physician is address the medical concerns as my patients present them. I hear their stories of illness, how they understand their perceived problems. I conduct a physical examination. I recollect bits and pieces and, sometimes, entire wholes of information I have learned, of facts and theories and patterns, and reconstruct them in my own mind focusing on the specific and particular needs of the person or people before me. I diagnose. I treat. I do what physicians of whatever ilk do: I attend to my patients' needs as best I can.

In response to those needs, I play many roles: interpreter, guide, diagnostician, advocate, and healer. In playing any one of these roles, I am supported by the structure, the knowledge, and the language I learned many years ago in medical school and residency. I am supported as well as by the titles I have earned, first as physician and later as family physician. But while my medical training continues to provide a framework for my work, it has been but a start to something more whole, more complete, and more authentic – to that which I truly treasure – my work as I see it, as a family doctor.

Conclusion

I am not oblivious to, nor have I been immune to, the difficulties that family physicians (or other primary care clinicians) face in today's medical environment. I certainly know that there are days when my family practice is not so joyful, when things go wrong, when mistakes are made, and when people (patients and professionals alike) are difficult to reach or even refuse to join in. I am aware, too, that within family medicine there are those who will not be able to comprehend my insights into practice and may, perhaps, even be threatened by them. But in writing this, I have chosen to hold up for inspection the fulfillment that my work brings to me. Rather than focus on the challenges of my work as a family doctor, some due to a socioeconomic structure that has fostered the creation of a medical industrial complex and others to the human need for conservatism and conformity,[20,21] I have chosen here to explore and appreciate the sources of that happiness and what continues to nurture it.

For it is in this exploration and appreciation that I am best able to find the gratification and satisfaction that Lynn Carmichael shared with me many years ago. It is by examining the myriad facets of my daily work, modest as they are meaningful, that I am able to sustain myself in contentment as a family physician. It is in doing this that I open myself – and my patients – to joy. So may we all.

References

1. Carmichael L. Voices from family medicine: Lynn Carmichael. Interview by William B. Ventres and John J. Frey. *Fam Med*. 1992; 24(1): 53–57.
2. Frey JJ. "Who is going to take care of the people?" Lynn Carmichael and his times. *Fam Med*. 2009; 41(8): 552–54.
3. Candib LM. *Medicine and the Family*. New York, NY: Basic Books; 1995.
4. Loxterkamp D. A vow of connectedness: views from the road to Beaver's farm. *Fam Med*. 2001; 33(4): 244–47.
5. Frey JJ III. Building our sense of place. *Fam Med*. 1998; 30(6): 401–03.
6. McWhinney I, Freeman T. *A Textbook of Family Medicine*. 3rd ed. New York, NY: Oxford University Press; 2009.
7. Berger J. *A Fortunate Man*. New York, NY: Vintage; 1997.
8. Turabian JL. Perez Franco B. El efecto de ver por primera vez el mar. Un intento de definición de la Ley Generalde la medicina de familia: La entrevista es la clínica [The effect of seeing the sea for the first time. An attempt at defining the family medicine law: the interview is clinical medicine]. *Aten Primaria*. 2008; 40(11): 565–66.
9. Blasco PG, Levites MR, Janaudis MA, et al. Family medicine education in Brazil: challenges, opportunities, and innovations. *Acad Med*. 2008; 83(7): 684–90.
10. Presno Labrador C. El médico de familia en Cuba [The family physician in Cuba]. *Rev Cubana Med Gen Integr*. 2006; 22(1). http://scielo.sld.cu/scielo.php?script=sci_arttext&pid=S0864-21252006000100015&lng=en (accessed May 23, 2011).
11. Paz O, Kemp L translator. *The Labyrinth of Solitude: Life and Thought in Mexico*. New York, NY: Grove Press; 1961. p. 42.
12. Ventres WB. Cultural encounters and family medicine: six lessons from South America. *J Am Board Fam Pract*. 1997; 10(3): 232–36.
13. Epstein RM. Mindful practice. *JAMA*. 1999; 282(9): 833–39.
14. McPhee SJ. The practice of presence. Presented at: *Alpha Omega Alpha Honor Society Spring Lecture*; April 17, 1981; Piscataway, NJ.
15. Rogers C. *On Becoming a Person*. Boston, MA: Houghton Mifflin Company; 1961.
16. Gabbard GO. The role of compulsiveness in the normal physician. *JAMA*. 1985; 254(20): 2926–29.

17. Brody H, Sparks HV Jr., Abbett WS, Wood DL, Wadland WC, Smith RC. The mammalian medical center for the 21st century. *JAMA*. 1993; 270(9): 1097–1100.

18. Engel GL. How much longer must medicine's science be bound by a seventeenth century world view? In: White KL. *The Task of Medicine: Dialogue at Wickenburg*. Menlo Park, CA: The Henry J. Kaiser Family Foundation; 1988. pp. 113–36.

19. Ferrer RL. A piece of my mind: within the system of no-system. *JAMA*. 2001; 286(20): 2513–14.

20. Starr P. *The Social Transformation of American Medicine*. New York, NY: Basic Books; 1982.

21. Coulehan J, Williams PC. Conflicting professional values in medical education. *Camb Q Healthc Ethics*. 2003; 12(1): 7–20.

5

Success, Regret, and the Struggle for Balance

Joseph A. Carrese, MD, MPH,
and Michel A. Ibrahim, MD, PhD

IN A ROLE REVERSAL, I ASKED MY PERSONAL PHYSICIAN, JOE, WHO IS A mid-career faculty member, "How are you doing?" And he replied, "Oh, I'm fine, but trying to balance career and family is not easy. I juggled my schedule a few weeks ago so I could teach a course to medical students in the evening – a time of the day that I usually reserve for my family. As it turned out, my daughter's high school soccer team made it to the regional finals, and the game was scheduled at the same time as the course. This created a major conflict for me: teach this special class (which is partly about balance in your life!) or attend my daughter's soccer game."

This conversation triggered some painful memories for me. I graduated from medical school about the time when Joe was born, and I was excessively driven to achieve professionally: I became a full professor before I was 40 years old and attained high-level administrative positions, including becoming dean of a large school at a prestigious university early in my career. But at what price? Following the lead of my colleagues and mentors of that era, I achieved this success at the expense of my personal and family life.

In recent times, attitudes have changed a bit. Younger physicians, particularly women, are trying to structure their careers so they have sufficient time for family life, in some cases by working part-time. Some physicians – both men and women – switch to fields with more flexible schedules, such as public health, preventive medicine, or other non-patient-care fields. But what about physicians who want to stay in clinical or academic medicine and strike a different balance between career and the rest of their lives? Can our institutions accommodate these people? Or must we conclude that they can't be successful at the highest levels?

The system I grew up in may not have changed that much during the past several decades. Institutions continue to be led by those (like me) who apply the same old rules of the game, and younger physicians are expected, for the most part, to follow along. Certainly, there are some who are remarkable in their ability to be meaningfully engaged in their kids' and their partners' lives and still achieve tremendous career success. Yet, for many, this approach, even if attainable, misses the point. Many younger faculty simply want more time with their families, particularly as they are raising their children. Regardless of approach, for most faculty real choices are required. Those who elect to commit less than the full measure of their time and energies to their career may not be able to succeed at the same pace and to the same level as in years past. And faculty who continue to allow their choices to be driven predominantly by institutional expectations and career-focused considerations are at risk for suffering the same personal losses I experienced.

Joe inquired whether anyone who was senior to me earlier in my career handled this balancing act differently. "Was there anyone who raised questions about this or made different choices?" he asked. I answered: "Very rarely!" I found myself recalling, with a feeling of dis-ease, a story I heard of a daughter who left a note in her drawer when she went away to college, telling her father that over the years he had sacrificed his family for the sake of his medical practice and had thus stolen something from her own life.

If I could turn the clock back, I would be content with becoming a professor later in life and not holding high administrative posts – if the trade-offs were not to go through a painful divorce and to have had better relationships with my kids. Because of the time I spent away from home while the children were growing up, it has not always been easy to communicate and to find common ground. They have almost never sought my advice on matters important to them, and rarely would they say "we learned this from you." Our relationships have not been what they might have been had we bonded while they were young. This is hindsight, of course, and neither does it presume a cause and effect, nor does it mean I would have done things differently at the time. (Now that my children have children of their own and I have a loving wife, our interactions have improved tremendously all around.)

I then asked: "How about you? Are you willing to trade off, honestly?" He answered: "I have – I basically already have. I'm 49 and I'm an associate professor, and I'm on a different career trajectory from many of my peers. Of course, one could argue that this may be more a reflection of my capabilities than any choices I've made about balance in my life. But I think it is possible that I would be further along in my career if I had made different choices. I have two teenage kids, and it has not been my experience as a father that I want or need to spend less time with them now than when they were infants or toddlers or younger children. If anything, I'm spending more time with them. My weekends are filled with their activities. It is wonderful, but there is a trade-off. I have chosen to be more selective about how frequently I travel and to where, and to coordinate these decisions with what's going on at home. But if I miss national meetings or decline to take on additional projects, that comes at a price. I'm perfectly willing to accept whatever career outcome follows from these choices. But I have to say that it is not easy making such choices, which are counter to institutional expectations and the existing reward system."

"What is success and how much achievement is enough?" I wondered. "People who have millions of dollars want more millions, but how many millions do you really need? The same applies to academic achievement – how many publications are enough for an institutional committee to recommend promotion?" Joe responded, "There are criteria, of course. But really, everybody has to answer that for themselves. For me, the answer to how many papers is enough is whatever I can do given the choices I've made about my time and priorities."

There will always be people who follow the model of continuous, relentless work to achieve at a potentially great cost to personal and family life. There are others who are happy with a moderate amount of career success, so they may attend to other domains in their lives. Our academic institutions need to be flexible and accommodate more than one approach. They need to recognize a new reality with respect to work-life issues, and they need to reflect that recognition in meaningful ways, such as acknowledging the legitimacy of part-time careers and rewarding faculty accordingly. Criteria for advancement could take into account whether a faculty member is working full time when reviewing his or her accomplishments, allowing for all faculty to be valued and rewarded fairly. We certainly have seen examples of this sort of flexibility from the corporate world.

I believe that many colleagues in my generation look with admiration at younger physicians, such as Joe, who are trying to balance a career in academic medicine with their personal life. At least I can speak for myself: I wish I had known better and exercised the option of spending more time with my family. I think that my colleagues would also envy the new generation's attitude about life and living. I think many of us wish that we had been able to do that, but at the time, we were following our role models. Now, although it is too late for me to make such choices, there are role models like Joe who will influence the younger generation to do it differently.

6

The Company We Keep

Why Physicians Should Refuse to See Pharmaceutical Representatives

Howard Brody, MD, PhD

Introduction

A majority of medical practitioners spend part of their time talking with and receiving gifts from pharmaceutical sales representatives (reps). Asked why they do so, most would initially be puzzled at the question. It is very likely that they have come to this place as a result of long-standing habit rather than conscious choice. Nonetheless, the decision to spend one's time in this fashion has important ethical implications. I will offer an ethical analysis and approach the analysis by way of the following analogy.

A Fanciful Analogy

Suppose I have an alcohol problem. Overall, I am making a fairly good recovery, but occasionally I fall off the wagon. In the past year, I have gotten drunk four times, each time while in the company of my friend Judy. Judy herself seldom drinks to excess; it is just that somehow, when I am in her company, I seem to lose the restraints that otherwise control my own drinking. Judy cheerfully rejects any suggestion that my drinking is her fault. I am an adult and can do what I like, she says.

I have many friends. Judy is not one of my closest friends, even though our acquaintance goes back a long way. Whatever I can do with Judy I could easily do with any number of other friends.

Now suppose that I say that I am deeply committed to remaining free of alcohol. Yet at the same time I insist that I will not give up seeing Judy and spending time in her company. How seriously do you take my protestations of yearning for sobriety?

This analogy may illuminate the ethical question of whether physicians should spend a portion of their time interacting with pharmaceutical reps. The more formal way of putting the argument is:

1. As a matter of professional integrity, I claim that I ought to behave in accord with certain principles.
2. Empirical evidence shows that I am highly likely to behave in ways contrary to my professional principles when I keep company with certain people.
3. My professional responsibilities do not require me to keep company with those people.
4. If, therefore, I choose to continue to keep company with those people, I cannot claim that I truly wish to adhere to those professional principles.

Ethical and Prudential Arguments

Ethical arguments about the relationship between individual physicians and reps have often been stated badly or at least incompletely. Those opposing cozy relationships often speak as if the reps are evil people or are guilty of moral wrongdoing. Standard arguments also portray physicians as akin to putty in the hands of the reps. This portrayal elicited a rebuttal that appeared in the *Wall Street Journal* in response to an article about a campaign by medical students to banish reps from teaching hospitals – that these arguments cast reps "as schemers with more money than sense and doctors as easily manipulated marionettes."[1]

The more complete argument is to see the issue as an interplay of ethical and prudential considerations. The prudential considerations have to do with how we as physicians elect to spend our time, given that almost all of us agree that we are extremely busy and work under tremendous time pressure. The ethical issue has to do with what professional duties we owe our patients. I will assume that the most important ethical duty is a commitment to serving the interests of the patient and avoiding potential conflicts that might divert one from that commitment.[2,3] A secondary ethical duty is to clinical competence, which includes accepting well-grounded medical evidence as the correct basis for one's actions.

The goal of the pharmaceutical industry is to increase its profits, which includes persuading physicians to prescribe more of the most expensive drugs.

Continually rising drug costs are not in the interests of our patient population as a whole, and the most expensive or most heavily marketed drug may not be the best prescription for any given patient. In a capitalist society the industry (I will assume) has every right to act this way, and pharmaceutical reps are honest business persons earning their salaries by serving their employers' interests. The existence of a potential conflict of interest with the physician of integrity need not imply that the drug industry is acting wrongly, merely that its goals are at least somewhat different from the goals of ethical medical practice. But when does a potential conflict become an actual conflict?

The Empirical Data

A few years ago my argument could not have been made in a convincing way about physicians and reps. Those skeptical about overly friendly relationships with the pharmaceutical industry could claim that accepting gifts from reps would very likely compromise the physician's integrity and clinical judgment, but few empirical data existed to prove that this actually happened. More recently, the available data have grown and have spoken unequivocally.

As long as a decade ago, physician leaders within a hospital were shown to be both heavily influenced by free trips to resorts at which they received pitches from reps and oblivious to the fact that they had been so influenced.[4] More recently, systematic reviews of the literature confirmed a direct relationship between the frequency of contact with reps and the likelihood that physicians will behave in ways favorable to the pharmaceutical industry.[5,6] Physicians who spend more time with reps are less likely to prescribe rationally.[7] Patients with hypertension that is treated with "free" drug samples are less likely to have their hypertension controlled than are patients whose hypertension is treated by the physicians' free choice of drugs.[8] Yet physicians influenced by pharmaceutical marketing nonetheless believe that their information is scientific and unbiased.[9,10]

The evidence available today, therefore, seems conclusive on 2 points – first, that we are indeed heavily influenced by reps; and second, that we ourselves are very poor judges of the extent of that influence.[10] To the extent that we claim to be scientific practitioners, we would seem obligated to take this evidence into account in deciding upon our proper professional behavior.

Using One's Time Wisely

Having accepted the ethical principles and the empirical data, the next question is one of prudence or efficiency – how to spend our time, assuming we want to maximize those professional values and also accept the validity of the data. Would a physician, under those circumstances, agree to spend time seeing reps?

Two aspects of the visit with the rep are receiving gifts (ranging from trinkets such as pens and notepads all the way to tickets to attend continuing education conferences in plush vacation spots) and learning information about the drugs sold by that company. There is some evidence that receiving gifts makes the physician more likely to feel a sense of debt to the company or the rep and therefore more likely to do their bidding.[10,11] If this were not so, the most profitable industry in the world is throwing about $13 billion annually down the drain.[12] So adherence to professional values – fidelity to the interests of the patient – would seem presumptively to dictate that one should not accept any gifts from reps.

What about listening to them present information? There is no empirical evidence to show what happens when reps present information only, with no exchange of gifts. It appears the gift exchange is such a basic part of the reps' armamentarium that one is simply never encountered without the other. Available evidence suggests nonetheless that information presented by the pharmaceutical industry is substantially biased in favor of the sponsor's product.[13,14] A dedicated and conscientious physician might therefore decide that it was consistent with his professional obligations to listen to drug reps (even perhaps professionally obligatory, on the assumption that one might first learn a useful bit of information from that source). It would then seem a necessary step that the physician immediately devote additional time to a careful search of the medical literature, or consultation with unbiased and evidence-based data sources, to double-check any information received, given that the bias of the reps' presentation is obvious and unavoidable.

To the best of my knowledge, few if any physicians who claim the "right" to see reps and to listen to their pitches actually spend the time necessary to research the information received and to correct for bias. These physicians then appear to be in a situation similar to the alcohol-challenged person in my example. If they choose to spend time in the company of the reps, where the data show unequivocally that they will encounter serious bias, and then refuse to spend the time needed to correct for that bias, how can they claim to adhere to the professional values of fidelity to the interests of the patient? On the other hand, imagine that the physician was sufficiently diligent to take the time needed to check on all the reps' statements. That physician would seem guilty of a serious time management problem. Surely if one were taking all that time independently to research pharmaceuticals, one need not spend any further time to meet with reps at all. Why divert that additional time away from patient care? Given how busy the average physician claims to be, could this use of one's time truly be the most efficient?[15]

The obvious rejoinder is that meeting with the reps is fun because they are friendly people and know precisely how to stroke physicianly egos, and they give out nice gifts.[15] This means, incidentally, that the analogy to the recovering alcoholic was not as far-fetched as it may have seemed. Spending time with reps and seeking their handouts are akin to an addiction. Medical students and residents are carefully seduced into this habit long before they become practitioners.[16] In this case, however, the reasons for meeting with them are purely personal, not professional, and should not be justified by any presumed claims toward professional education or service. One sees one's golfing buddies outside office hours.

An Objection

My argument could be claimed to fall apart with its premise[3]: My professional responsibilities do not require me to keep company with those people. The rejoinder is: My professional responsibility requires that I try my best to serve my indigent patients, which in turn means keeping a generous stock of free samples, and I can do so only by seeing the reps and listening to their pitches.

In some medical settings I believe the rejoinder is persuasive. My colleague the wound surgeon, for example, can treat his poor nursing home patients with severe decubiti only by applying very expensive products, which he can obtain as samples from the reps, but which would be prohibitively expensive if he tried to purchase them himself for the patients. Some primary care physicians with overwhelmingly low-income practices might be in similar straits.

In the more usual practice setting, however, there are several problems with the rejoinder. First, many samples never reach indigent patients but instead go home with the physicians and office staff.[17] (Other samples go to well-off patients as a matter of convenience, not need.) Second, if the average primary care group were to stock the sample cupboard with generic drugs that are used to treat the most frequently encountered problems in their practice, the cost of the drugs would be well within their means to pay for out of practice or personal funds.[18] A generic drug sample cupboard would save them from starting treatment with an expensive drug because a free sample was handy, and then having the patient remain on an irrational or expensive drug simply because it is easier to prescribe again rather than to start anew with a more sensible alternative.[19] Westfall, in arguing why family physicians should avoid seeing reps, argued that there is almost always a superior way to secure needed drugs for indigent patients other than to rely on samples.[20]

Conclusion

Reps are not evil, but they are time-consuming and serve interests that often are at odds with those of our patients. To spend time with reps in a manner that preserves professional integrity would require both refusing to accept their gifts and spending a great deal of valuable time double-checking their information. I propose that the vast majority of physicians could spend their time in better ways.

Lately everyone seems to be concerned about our ethical integrity. The pharmaceutical companies themselves announced with great fanfare in 2002 a new code of ethics that would limit the more outrageous gifts.[21] The Federal government later that year announced investigations into whether some gift-giving schemes violated anti-kickback laws.[22] The American College of Physicians issued stricter guidelines for individual physicians.[23]

Despite these authoritative pronouncements, the drug rep habit has proved extremely difficult to break. As far back as 1961, thoughtful physicians made the same ethical arguments that one hears today, apparently with little effect during the interim.[24] Two reasons for our resistance to this ethical message may be that our medical culture stresses a sense of entitlement to reps' goodies and that we have an apparently endless ability to rationalize why we see reps and accept their gifts while imagining we are little influenced as a result.[10,15]

One further ethical analysis is hardly likely to produce a sea change in our attitudes and behavior when this change has been so difficult to produce previously. Nonetheless, I remain hopeful that stressing the prudential time-management aspect of the problem might catch the attention of some of us who are otherwise resistant to the message. Given how busy most of us are, it seems increasingly hard to defend a practice that further robs us of valuable time.

As important as time management is, one would still wish that our profession cared even more about professional integrity and commitment to the well-being of our patients. Reps are honest business people, mostly, who have no power over our professional integrity; it belongs to us. Once we are firmly committed to regaining our integrity, we will have no trouble deciding that it is worth more to us than any number of pens, coffee mugs, and sandwiches.

References

1. Sebra J. Drug reps and doctors took an undeserved hit. *Wall Street Journal*. July 12, 2002: A9.
2. Rothman DJ. Medical professionalism – focusing on the real issues. *N Engl J Med*. 2000; 342: 1283–86.

3. Schafer A. Biomedical conflicts of interest: a defence of the sequestration thesis-learning from the cases of Nancy Olivieri and David Healy. *J Med Ethics*. 2004; 30: 8–24.
4. Orlowski JP, Wateska L. The effects of pharmaceutical firm enticements on physician prescribing patterns. There's no such thing as a free lunch. *Chest*. 1992; 102: 270–73.
5. Wazana A. Physicians and the pharmaceutical industry: is a gift ever just a gift? *JAMA*. 2000; 283: 373–80.
6. Reviews: What impact does pharmaceutical promotion have on behavior? Drug Promotion Database. Available at: http://apps.who.int/medicinedocs/pdf/s8109e/s8109e.pdf.
7. Figueiras A, Caamano F, Gestal-Otero JJ. Influence of physician's education, drug information and medical-care settings on the quality of drugs prescribed. *Eur J Clin Pharmacol*. 2000; 56: 747–53.
8. Zweifler J, Hughes S, Schafer S, et al. Are sample medicines hurting the uninsured? *J Am Board Fam Pract*. 2002; 15: 361–66.
9. Avorn J, Chen M, Hartley R. Scientific versus commercial sources of influence on the prescribing behavior of physicians. *Am J Med*. 1982; 73: 4–8.
10. Dana J, Loewenstein G. A social science perspective on gifts to physicians from industry. *JAMA*. 2003; 290: 252–55.
11. Chren MM, Landefeld CS, Murray TH. Doctors, drug companies, and gifts. *JAMA*. 1989; 262: 3448–451.
12. Rosenthal MB, Berndt ER, Donahue JM, et al. Promotion of prescription drugs to consumers. *N Engl J Med*. 2002; 346: 498–505.
13. Ziegler MG, Lew P, Singer BC. The accuracy of drug information from pharmaceutical sales representatives. *JAMA*. 1995; 273: 1296–98.
14. Murphy S. Gifts seen as effective by drug company reps. *Boston Globe*. Nov. 17, 2002: B1.
15. Griffith D. Reasons for not seeing drug representatives. *BMJ*. 1999; 319: 69–70.
16. Kassirer JP. A piece of my mind: financial indigestion. *JAMA*. 2000; 284: 2156–57.
17. Westfall JM, McCabe J, Nicholas RA. Personal use of drug samples by physicians and office staff. *JAMA*. 1997; 278: 141–43.
18. Erickson S. Closing the sample closet: How well could you get along without medication samples--and without drug reps? Very well, according to the authors. *Fam Pract Management*. 1995; 2: 43–47.
19. Chew LD, O'Young TS, Hazlet TK, et al. A physician survey of the effect of drug sample availability on physicians' behavior. *J Gen Intern Med*. 2000; 15: 478–83.
20. Westfall JM. Physicians, pharmaceutical representatives, and patients: who really benefits? *J Fam Pract*. 2000; 49: 817–19.
21. Hensley S. Sorry, Doc, no dinners-to-go: drug sales reps begin building a new marketing playbook. *Wall Street Journal*. April 23, 2002:D4.
22. Pear R. Drug industry is told to stop gifts to doctors. *New York Times*. Oct. 1, 2002:A1.
23. Coyle SL. Physician-industry relations. Part 1: individual physicians. *Ann Intern Med*. 2002: 136: 396–402.
24. May CD. Selling drugs by "educating" physicians. *J Med Educ*. 1961; 36: 1–23.

7

Doctors' Work

Eulogy for My Vocation

David Loxterkamp, MD

What the world needs is people who have come alive.

—Howard Thurman[1]

I DON'T REMEMBER IT SLIPPING AWAY, ONLY THE SHIVER OF CERTAINTY it was gone. A personal calling – the vocation to medicine – was my collateral deposit on a career that promised both conviction and sense of fulfillment. Now it was scattered like the lofted pieces of a jigsaw puzzle. What remained was the gift to see my work differently, less chiseled in stone or latched to some sacred destiny.

It is hard for a cradle Catholic to discount the pledges recited on graduate day – the Prayer of Maimonides, the Oath of Hippocrates, the Declaration of Geneva. They are grave, ethereal, and lasting. One is fashioned to be a doctor, not trained to meet performance standards. One is chosen forever, not certified or employed for the length of the contract. One is vowed to the life-long pursuit of perfection. When all this was cast into doubt, I did not rush to the dark side. Work has remained more than a meal ticket, servility to a role, contractual obligation, or family tradition. It is a work in progress, as much defined by those I care for as by those who labor beside me.

Giovanni

An old artist came to see me. He reported that his creative juices had run dry. He could no longer sculpt and, as a result, had trouble maintaining his income and reputation. It had been better for him at University, where he taught for many years. There he had a train of admiring students, made regular rounds on the lecture circuit, and married a younger woman when their difference in age was more flattering than problematic. Then, as if overnight, he began to see himself as old, forgotten, and ineffectual, even in the bedroom where he once prided himself to be the master.

Diagnoses ran through my mind. I knew which tests to order, the drugs I might prescribe. As Giovanni railed against his misfortune, tears welled in his eyes … and mine. I sensed that something more was at stake: a tug at my own self-confidence, the gravitational pull on the arc of my career.

We make choices. We are boxed by our abilities and temperament. We are caught in currents stronger and deeper than we dare to imagine. To paraphrase Freud, the important decisions of personal life are governed by the deep inner needs of our nature.[2]

Parallel Professions

My partners and I recently gave up our hospital privileges "to focus on other interests," I often felt it necessary to add. But honestly, I was tired of the scrutiny, the liability, the bureaucracy, and after-hours call. And there was plenty of work to do in the office, where the pace and personalities were more to my liking. Yet doubts arose: Could I afford to slow down? Would I lose professional respect? Was I more than the sum of my diminishing parts?

I had been preparing for a career in medicine since fifth grade. A wrinkled photograph shows me dressed as a country doctor for the Rolfe, Iowa, Centennial Parade. My father – a GP – provided the props, which I would later inherit upon his sudden death. The new specialty of family practice hooked me with the promise of caring for the disenfranchised, and my Catholic upbringing assured me that I had a calling.

But I was called too often. Away from my wife and kids. Away from the self-satisfaction of enjoying a job well done, or reflecting on the deep inner needs of my nature. At mid-career, the shelter of a vocation was splintered by the prophetic words of Howard Thurman, "Don't ask what the world needs. Ask what makes you come alive, and go do it. Because what the world needs is people who have come alive."[1]

So I have softened my mistrust (and envy) of younger colleagues who changed the rules, took the more competitive offer, and worked part-time in order to parent and pursue other interests. They still face the age-old challenge: how to put food on the table and get ahead without worshipping the gods of consumption and achievement. Nor do I disparage those who wear their profession like a suit of armor. Let's eulogize our differences, not bury them, and talk of the deep dimensions of our lives.

Amateurs

The old sculptor belonged to our wider circle of friends, so it did not surprise me when we met again at a dinner party. The conversation soon turned to careers and the challenges faced by aging professionals. "Too much competition," he pined; "everyone claims to be an artist these days without life experience, or training, or the self-discipline to create nuanced and dialectic art." Or, as he saw it, real art. Admittedly, this logic was the loaded gun I once brandished against midlevel and holistic practitioners.

Then, by way of analogy, I waded into a minefield of my own. The professional ball player and sandlot amateur, I argued, share much in common. Both love the game and strive for personal glory, self-improvement, and peer acceptance through their sport. But there is an essential difference, more poignant than salary. It is the difference between having a vocation or an avocation. For the major league player and most professionals, work becomes their identity.

Eventually my friend may see his career as more than reputation, salary, portfolio, influence, or lasting contribution. His work is also teamwork. It is meant to please his fans. Work is our open door, our best shot at feeling fully connected, loved, and a servant for others. He, like the rest of us, may see his work as a means to an end. Or come to believe that feelings of connection and love flow from who we are, not from what we do. They stem from an inner nature that cannot be taken away from us or exhausted in our fervor to bestow it.

I look to you, Giovanni, and ponder the 10 years that precede my retirement, just as you reflect on a decade hence. We cannot repair the crumbling pillars of our faith, whatever the convictions we once held. Nor can they be easily replaced. You must know that the idea of vocation has been a struggle for me, too. This Catholic, this orphan, this good and able child who fell far short in earning the love he desperately sought. I am learning the art of tolerance, tolerance especially for the sorrow, longing, and imperfections that have taken up permanent residence inside me.

We are not the only ones who worry about a legacy. Every day I listen to patients who lament their lost dreams and the cruel twists of fate. Yet somehow we are all surviving, helped – I believe – by a mutual desire for honest conversation.

This is my life's real work, the great corpus, the body that I and so many of my colleagues offer the patient in unremarkable ways. It is, of course, our own body – just us – sitting behind closed doors with another who is equally muddled or maimed. Another who – to our joy and surprise – is able to come alive.

References

1. Thurman H. *With Head and Heart: The Autobiography of Howard Thurman*. Chicago: Harvest/HBJ Book, 1981.
2. Masson JM. The Complete Letters of Sigmund Freud to Wilhelm Fliess, 1887–1904 (1985). Cambridge, MA and London, England: The Belknap Press of Harvard University Press; 1985.

Section 2

Patient Care and Caring

A seemingly endless number of standardized guidelines are available to help clinicians treat diseases and provide preventive services. However, caring for patients – whole people with accomplishments and flaws – is rarely a standardized process. In primary care, encounters are shaped by patients, with their unique life stories, and physicians, who "[welcome] the richness and the complexity of the complete human being"[1] and then tailor care to that person's distinct health care needs.[2]

In this section, we explore personalized approaches to patient care as we meet an array of characters.

- *Sally*, Dean Gianakos's feisty elderly patient, who reminds us that treating a patient does not always mean treating a medical condition.
- *The Old Duffers' Club*, whose members helped David Loxterkamp learn to care for the elderly by slowing down, connecting, and attending to the details of daily living; as we age, a sense of purpose and an ordinary life are our anchors.
- *Family physician Steven Landers*, who finds satisfaction and meaning in caring for patients in their homes. He sits with them and listens – a compassionate guest – as he strives to provide personal and relevant care.
- *Henry*, who is stuck in a medical system that treats diseases rather than people. Richard Allen recounts a young physician's attempts to cheer a patient who simply wants to be left alone.
- *Thomas Bodenheimer's left foot*: when a physician and researcher of chronic disease experiences his own chronic condition, he learns that tending to emotional and mental suffering is an inextricable part of physical healing.

References

1. Mullan F. *Big Doctoring in America: Profiles in Primary Care*. Berkeley: University of California Press; 2002. p. xi.
2. Stange KC, Jaén CR, Flocke SA, et al. The value of a family physician. *J Fam Pract*. 1998; 46(5): 363–68.

8

Pounds

Dean Gianakos, MD

LIKE MANY DOCTORS, I HAVE THE UNFORTUNATE HABIT OF SCANNING my office schedule to see which patients will make or break my day. This morning, I'm happy to see Sally's name on the list. She waves to me as Anne escorts her into an examination room. A few minutes later, I walk into the room and notice the large plastic bag at her feet. Before I can say hello, Sally pulls two boxes from the bag.

"Fifty-one," she says proudly. "Make that 52. Here's one for you, and one for Anne."

"Fifty-two?" I ask.

"Don't look so surprised, doc. I baked 52 of 'em over the holidays. Lemon pound, chocolate layer, apple-orange, and a few other favorites."

Last visit she brought me the best lemon pound cake I'd ever tasted, and I let her know many times. Sally's cakes are so good my colleagues tease me about having her return to the office every month! In truth, she comes in only when she is sick.

"You're pretty amazing," I tell her.

"So are you."

She has been entertaining 30 people at her house every Sunday afternoon for the past 50 years. Ham, turkey, vegetables, and pound cake for everybody.

"Okay, Sally. Don't tell me. You've been coughing and wheezing for the past 2 weeks."

She smiles.

"You've also run out of your inhalers. You're waking up at night coughing and carrying on. You're here today because you're worried you won't have enough wind to make Sunday dinner. Did I leave anything out?"

"No, that's about right."

We both laugh. We both laugh because it's the same story every time she comes in, and I know it well. When I was younger, I used to reproach Sally about her noncompliant behavior. She never gave me her reasons. After years of caring for her, I now understand: it's about pride, a tight budget, and her unwillingness to entertain the concept of prevention. It's also about my own inability to follow a strict, medical regimen (i.e., reduce my fat intake).

"Hop up here," I tell her.

She climbs on the examination table with ease. As I examine her, I playfully scold her about waiting until the last minute to come in. "Pick up the phone," I tell her. "Call me. Call Anne." Again, she prefers to tough it out.

I hear wheezes throughout her lungs.

"You get this prednisone filled as soon as you leave here."

"Yes sir," she barks out, in the middle of a cough.

"And here are a few steroid inhalers (remember these?) to keep your asthma in check."

Of course, whom am I fooling? She never uses her steroid inhalers.

"They don't work like the other ones," she says, "and besides, why should I take them when I normally feel so good?"

How do you feel now, I want to say. On second thought, no sense getting upset about it. Not much I can teach a spunky, 91-year-old woman about how to live her life.

As I slice another piece of lemon pound cake, I muse, "High-fat snack. Cholesterol 245 mg/dL last week. Remember what the scale showed this morning?"

"True, but I'd hate to disappoint Sally!"

9

The Old Duffers' Club

David Loxterkamp, MD

> *Ordinariness is the most precious thing we struggle for ... the right
> to go on living with a sense of purpose and a sense of self-worth – an
> ordinary life.*
>
> —Irena Klepfisz[1]

THEY COME EVERY TWO WEEKS, ON SNOW-PACKED ROADS OR UNDER
aquiline skies, often an hour early and sometimes a day late. But faithfully they
come: the six founding members of the Elder Men's Education and Support
Group. They gather with serious intent for friendship and conversation around
a narrow circle of chairs in a tiny conference room at the far end of my office.
They take a chance that to merely disclose their particular circumstance, their
isolation and loneliness, will help them face their uncertain future.

The idea for what became known as The Old Duffers' Club sprang from the
confluence of a week in practice: five elderly patients – retired teachers, business-
men, mechanics, pipe-fitters – confessed their feelings of uselessness and loss
of direction. One gentleman, a wiry, soft-spoken, independent Mainer, struck a
resonant chord:

> "How are you, Harold? What's happened since the last time we sat down?"
>
> "Well, Doc, I just returned from a moose hunt. I won a stamp in the lottery
> and shared it with my son and his friend. We got our moose, but [he glanced
> away] I wasn't much help in hauling it from the woods."
>
> I could hear a crack in his voice, as he swallowed hard on his words and

squeezed back tears. All the gentle coaxing, rephrasing, exploring of the logical angles could not flush out his feelings. Now, five minutes past our appointed time, I asked if he would return in a week to finish our conversation. He nodded yes, gathered himself up, and left without a word. When he returned a week later, he was still at a loss for what had washed over him.

"It's nothing, Doc. I've been a little teary since the stroke."

"Harold, whatever you are going through, you are not alone. I know there are others [soon to be discovered] who would sit down with you and see where it leads. Are you willing? Can I give you a call?"

During the next two weeks I jotted a list of potential candidates. Eleven men received my initial invitation, and eight attended the first organizational meeting. A final six settled into the regular conversations that became, soon enough, the ODC.

Slow Medicine

Long before, I had become aware of my failure to meet the needs of aging patients. The Old Duffers' Club provided a concrete corrective. But the larger gestalt required of our health care system is sweepingly outlined in Dennis McCullough's new book, *My Mother, Your Mother*.[2] Here he describes how "slow medicine" can help the elderly find or retain living conditions that will optimize the last years of their lives. Says McCullough, "Slow medicine is just this caring process of slowing down, being patient, coordinating care, and remaining faithful to the end. Families necessarily bear the greatest responsibility in surmounting [end of life] difficulties to create this bond of trust and security for their loved ones."

Contrast slow medicine with the brand of health care practiced in our emergency departments. Here a generation of specialists has been trained to react quickly, with increasing efficiency, using carefully constructed protocols, marshaling a mind-boggling array of resources to diagnose and intervene before a patient ever leaves their department. They have little or no foreknowledge of the individual; they have one chance to get it right. Because it is procedural, because it is crisis oriented, they have always enjoyed moral justification and reliable revenues for a system that, overall, produces underwhelming results. The problem lies neither in the training nor the protocol, but their application to all that inevitably floods the emergency department – too much of which is primary care.

McCullough's book is sprinkled with vignettes and powered by his personal experience as a geriatrician at Dartmouth Medical School and the Kendal-at-Hanover community of elders. He appeals to two groups of readers: doctors who are frustrated by the turnstile pace of ambulatory medicine, and families of the elderly who most of all need the ear, the patience, the clinical restraint, and careful watch of physicians who know them well. Rather than offer programmatic solutions, McCullough appeals to us personally. Kindness, he suggests, is the single most reliable ethical and practical guide to doing the work well. Preservation of function should be the priority of homes inhabited by the elderly so that their inevitable decline can be managed for as long as possible outside a nursing home.

McCullough resists the call for more professionals and better checklists to aid the war on aging. Instead, he encourages us to slow down and enlist families as we struggle to understand and address the needs of elderly neighbors and parents.

Mrs McGreavey lives up the street. Sitting on her rotting back porch with a yappy terrier leashed to the clothesline, she often waves to me as I jog past. Her son and daughter-in-law recently escorted her to an appointment with concerns about her memory. Indeed, she had not been seen in our office for over three years, a lapse in my memory, too. She complained of sleeping poorly, fearful that a 7- or 8-year-old boy had been entering her house and stealing cookies.

"Did you lock your door?"

"Of course, but he made an extra key."

"Could you change the lock?"

Her son hangs his head in frustration, having engaged the locksmith three times in the last six months.

"Why does he take only cookies, when there are other valuables in the home?"

"Truth be known, Dr Loxterkamp, he also steals my new brooms and leaves me with old, ragged ones."

She is so convincing, so sincere in her telling that I wonder if this mysterious boy is my son, a lover of cookies but decidedly allergic to dust and brooms.

"Have you seen the boy?"

"No."

"Then how do you know he is 7 or 8?"

"Because I know his mother. She's a nurse who lives across the street."

"Then why don't you ask her to give her son a stern talking to?"

"I don't know her name."

There is no dissuading her; the story rises above her inconsistencies. Dr McCullough is right: our worries for the patient often hover below the thresholds of the Mini Mental State Exam and depression inventory. Because this is

Mrs Greavey's annual exam, I order tests and set a time to review the results. Meanwhile, the son and I plan to enlist the community's resources and commit to closer surveillance in hopes of keeping my neighbor in her cozy house with the yappy dog for as long as possible.

Al and Roberta Pendleton have been my patients since I moved here a quarter-century ago. They are dead ringers for the couple in Grant Wood's famous painting American Gothic: silent, stoic, and standing by each other's side for more than 70 years. On the occasional home visit, one is always "doing fine" but "worried to death" about the other. Twenty years ago they might have moved out of their rambling farmhouse which – like themselves – was in need of repair. But the window of opportunity closed. The children anxiously shored up support. The son designed an expensive new addition and synchronized a rotation of home health aides that kept his parents at home a few months more before they died.

Despite our prayers for a quick and painless death, it will likely come by another route. We will follow that well-worn path from home to clinic, ambulance cot to hospital bed, rehabilitation facility to home care, and round the base paths again. Most of the crises that turn the wheel are predictable but unpreventable; many of the obvious safety nets choke the freedoms and desires of those we are trying to help. Denial is the preferred bullet for besting change. It thwarts children who otherwise exert their firm upper hand. It stymies doctors who think that clinical realities should dictate the better course. This long and uncertain drama requires time, tolerance, family allegiance, and an unbending desire to discover and place the patient's needs before our own.

Slow Change

How can we accomplish this in our own practices? I am not sure, and I am not there – yet. Here are ways we might begin:

- Individualize the ordering of mammograms, prostate cancer screening tests, Papanicolaou smears, or colonoscopies for anyone older than 80 years. Why measure cholesterol levels or bone density if the results don't alter our treatment? Increasingly, we do so to gild the quality assurance report and payment for performance, though there is little evidence that these tests matter in the elderly. For most, an annual breast examination, digital rectal examination, and stool occult blood test will suffice.
- Be attentive to the safety concerns of driving, balance, and memory loss. Inquire about alcohol consumption, daily nutrition, sleep habits, and regular

exercise. McCullough believes that compromised mobility is one of the most sensitive indicators of a person's well-being because it affects so many systems, from digestion, circulation, balance, and strength to overall emotional health.

- Advocate for necessary changes in the health care system that would reimburse us for unrushed office visits and family meetings. Reclaim our leadership role in home care, rather than relinquish it to agencies and aids. Fund research that specifically recruits the elderly and tests the intuition that less is more. Train hospitalists with a strong primary care orientation for the courage and wisdom to share important management decisions with patients and their physicians in the settings where they live.

- Focus on the little things that occupy our patients' lives, known by their acronym ADL, or activities of daily living. Advanced ADLs are the social skills that allow active participation in community life, including the ability to drive. Intermediate ADLs let us live independently in an apartment, requiring the ability to cook, houseclean, use the telephone, and pay bills. Basic ADLs are the skills of personal care – eating, dressing, bathing, and using the toilet. We sometimes forget that as a person's universe narrows, these simple tasks occupy monumental importance. I am reminded of this importance in the words of a Holocaust survivor, Irena Klepfisz, speaking on the 45th anniversary of the uprising of the Warsaw Ghetto:

> What we grieve for is not the loss of a grand vision, but rather the loss of common things, events and gestures. . . . Ordinariness is the most precious thing we struggle for, what the Jews of the Warsaw Ghetto fought for. Not noble causes or abstract theories. But the right to go on living with a sense of purpose and a sense of self-worth – an ordinary life.[1]

This is what is at stake for the elderly as friends die, functions fail, and independence slips away or is forced from their grasp.

Slow Talk

Which brings me back to the Old Duffers' Club.

What have we actually accomplished by our meetings? None of us claims to be working on a Master's of Duffer (MD) degree. A lucky few will realize the more elusive prize of *Duffer Ordinaire* (DO). This is, in fact, our ticket for admission:

that we are willing to acknowledge our age, commonality, and need for friendship. No group is smart enough, accomplished enough, or popular enough to please those who ride in on the high horse of pride.

At the first meeting, I asked each member what had drawn him there. Nearly all reported that they had lost a sense of direction and purpose. Two were widowers. One recently sold his life-long stamp collection; another gave up the clarinet. Each meeting began with a check-in, where we could discuss any event that involved us in the previous two weeks. There was one fellow, a retired professor, who uneasily confessed that he had done nothing except pass his empty hours in the recliner.

With time, the group began to talk of their activities. One wrote a letter to an old classmate, a best friend with whom he had lost contact. Another was planning a tour of the Western national parks. Still another came to terms with his eventual move out of state, where his younger wife had family and needed more of Grandma's time. It had now become their mutual decision, made for a hard but higher cause. And in recent weeks, the professor talked of taking his wife out to lunch, returned for lectures at Senior College, and suggested that the ODC meet at a restaurant for our final gathering before summer break. At that meal, I gave them each a gift, a T-shirt with the printed letters ODC and an image of the compass rose: symbol of their search for direction.

One of the Duffers caught me off guard recently when he asked, "Are you doing this group as much for yourself as for the rest of us?" Of course, I realized! Life is messy, purposes oblique, endings in doubt, and companionship essential. We are all looking more mercifully at our lives, knowing that many circumstances will not improve. Robin Sarah, in her poem "Tickets," provides insight on how people come to embrace the string of accidents that constitute a life. We are in a theater watching an unfamiliar play. When it is almost over, we realize that it was not the play we had purchased tickets for. We could leave – "some people do" – but feel compelled to stay "all through the tedious denouement to the unsurprising end – riveted, as it were; spellbound by our own imperfect lives, because they are lives."[3]

What have I learned from the old duffers? They are a grateful lot. They have no schemes for getting ahead, nor do they dwell in a photo-album past. They have only the present at their disposal and, in their vulnerability and loneliness, have learned to share it. Lack of direction and loss of purpose can be the price we pay for defaulting on society's standards of success. When wealth, fame, and productivity sift away, what remains is friendship. What remain are conversation, honesty, kindness, and affection. These are the tools well-used and well-kept by average people, the ones that William Stafford praises in his poem "Allegiances." While the hero travels to the mountaintop to capture his dreams, the rest of us can find comfort in the routines he left behind. In our doubts and restlessness, "we ordinary beings can cling to the earth and love where we are, sturdy for the common things."[4]

Ordinary lives are made extraordinary by this awareness. It is a lesson learned late, often too late for the likes of Mrs McGreavy. It is not too late for her family, Harold, the other members of the ODC, and their doctor. Slow medicine allows physicians to be a helpful part of end-of-life transitions. It makes it more likely that our patients will negotiate them successfully. There is only one club, claimed by all: why pretend otherwise? Let's toast our membership in the universal ODC. Teaching by example, let's slow down to a conversational pace, enjoy our simple dreams, and appreciate ordinary patients in need of the most ordinary brand of medicine, which is our primary care.

References

1. Keillor G. *The Writer's Almanac with Garrison Keillor*, American Public Media. Available at: http://writersalmanac.publicradio.org/index/php?date=2008/04/19.
2. McCullough D. *My Mother, Your Mother: Embracing Slow Medicine, the Compassionate Approach to Caring for Your Aging Loved Ones*. New York, NY: HarperCollins Publishers; 2008.
3. Sarah R. Riveted. In: *A Day's Grace: Poems 1997–2002*. Erin, Ontario: The Porcupine's Quill; 2003.
4. Stafford W. Allegiances. In: *The Darkness Around Us Is Deep: Selected Poems*. New York, NY: Harper Perennial; 1993.

10

Home Care

A Key to the Future of Family Medicine?

Steven H. Landers, MD, MPH

HE POPPED OUT THE FRONT DOOR, CAME DOWN THE ROTTING PORCH, and took the wrench from my hand. "A white man in a shirt and tie shouldn't be changin' a flat," he said. I awkwardly stepped back and wiped the sweat off my brow. He was a short black man in a well-worn navy blue mechanic's outfit, his baseball cap backwards with the rim flipped up. He came too close too quick and was laughing like he was drunk. I panned the block – vacant lot, boarded up house, cars passing, drivers staring. A young woman in tight blue shorts and a half-length top slowly walked past. He stared her down. "You all think every woman walkin' this street is hookin'," she said, and kept walking. She headed toward the corner store two blocks up, one of the "beer, lotto, cigarettes," places that are scattered throughout this part of town, where several people were standing.

This moment quickly became the most uncomfortable in my first three months on the job. I just finished my family medicine residency at Case Western Reserve University/University Hospitals of Cleveland in June, and I decided to stay on to help start a new house call/home primary care program. Our program is similar to others that have sprouted up around the country in recent years, possibly in response to the aging population and higher Medicare-allowable reimbursement for home visits.[1] I work closely with a nurse-practitioner, and we try and coordinate our care with home health companies and community aging agencies.

Fortunately, my car trouble has been limited to that single episode. There have been other inconveniences – it was a hot summer, most of my patients don't have air conditioners, and I'm a pretty big guy who easily sweats. The heat and sometimes the odors, such as the stench of tobacco and urine, can be unpleasant.

But, in many ways I have felt more comfortable doing home visits than I ever did in my residency continuity clinic. Though my medical school and residency training did not emphasize home care and house calls, I'm finding that the home is a natural place for our specialty. We have the social conscience to part with the comfort and familiarity of the office, we are trained to facilitate family problem solving, and we are a modern extension of the traditional generalist physicians that thrived in the home. As the United States seeks ways to address the health care needs of an aging population, elevating the role of family physicians in home care could be a satisfying intervention for both the health care system and physicians.

Most of my visits typically take 30 to 40 minutes, and it's hard not to linger a bit longer to talk about the weather, a book on the table, or a photograph on the wall. I'm learning very practical things about my patients, such as how they manage their medicines and diet, and I'm meeting family members and neighbors to enlist as a caregiving team who would not be present at an office visit. This deeper understanding of my patients has empowered me to provide more relevant – and likely more effective – preventive and chronic disease counseling and care coordination. Away from my office, as a guest in patients' homes, I am forced not to rush. Instead of standing above them, I usually must sit beside them on their couch or even on their bed, so we become closer. I've had more hugs and held more hands in three months than I did in three years. I feel like I'm caring for my patients and that they care for me.

The lectures about family dynamics, patient-centered care, and the community health curriculum are becoming more relevant, whereas just a few months ago in my residency continuity clinic, they didn't always add up in the 15-minute "get 'em in and out" clinic visits I was becoming accustomed to. In that world, I often dreaded a sick patient with multiple problems, family conflict, and dementia. The number of medications, unresolved issues, and consultants could make my head spin. These patients were too hard to fit into the clinic schedule. "Please let it be an introverted 30-year-old with a mild case of allergic rhinitis," I would sometimes think as I knocked on the door. I became a family doctor because I wanted to help people in need, but for me, those who were most needy and vulnerable became burdensome in 10- to 15-patient half-day sessions. Experiencing sick patients as burdensome was very unsatisfying, and feeling burdensome is likely unsatisfying for the patients, too. After waiting for a ride, spending sometimes hours in the waiting room, and leaving with unresolved concerns, patients and caregivers are often left to pick up the pieces at home through an automated telephone tree or, even worse, the emergency department.

According to the undercurrents I hear from students and colleagues, enthusiasm for high-volume office-based family medicine is waning. Clearly, our specialty is in transition, and the concerns I've raised are not new. Some are addressed in the Future of Family Medicine project report, and I'm optimistic that elements of the New Model will make family medicine offices more satis- fying places for doctors and patients.[2] I think the home could be another key to the future of family medicine. The US population of those older than 65 years is expected to grow to more than 70 million by 2030, and many will have physical and cognitive disabilities that make it difficult for them to leave their homes.[3] I believe the home is an ideal place to care for the most frail, most complex, and most costly older patients, and there are published studies that support this con- viction.[4–6] Family physicians working within multidisciplinary teams are ideal for this job. In light of recent downward trends of internal medicine resident interest in primary care and geriatrics training, there is an enormous opportunity for family physicians to rise up to meet this oncoming societal need.

In addition to providing better care in a more satisfying way, home care can be financially viable. In 1998 Medicare increased the allowable reimbursement for home visits by almost 50%. In 2005 the allowed charge for a detailed visit to an established patient was about $110.[7] Medicare also allows physicians to charge for home care plan certification and oversight for home-bound patients receiving nursing and rehabilitation services. Furthermore, although the volume of a home care practice is less than that of an office, the overhead is less. These factors appear to be influencing clinicians to provide more home care, as reflected by the rapid increase from 1998 to 2004 in the volume and charges for house calls.[1] By using miniature computers, cellular telephones, mobile imaging, port- able electrocardiograms, pulse oximeters, and other point-of-service diagnostics, the physician doesn't need to step backward from the technology of the modern medical practice.[8] Making house calls full time is not for everyone, but doing more than a token visit and putting an emphasis on home care may be possible for many practices.

In his 1997 Nicholas J. Pisacano Lecture, Ian McWhinney made an impas- sioned plea for family medicine to "return to our roots" by making home visits. McWhinney reminded us that, "The home is where the family's values are expressed," and that, "There is deep symbolism in the home visit…. It says 'I care enough about you to leave my power base … to come and see you on your own ground.' The symbolism is especially strong in the care of the dying."[9] In light of the aging population, advances in technology, and recent changes in Medicare reimbursement, this return to the home may now be possible. In fact, embracing home care may be a key part of the ongoing relevance and success of our specialty.

References

1. Landers SH, Gunn PW, Flocke SA, et al. Trends in house calls to Medicare beneficiaries. *JAMA*. 2005; 294: 2435–36.
2. Martin JC, Avant RF, Bowman MA, et al. The Future of Family Medicine: a collaborative project of the family medicine community. *Ann Fam Med*. 2004; 2(Suppl 1): S3–S32.
3. Besdine R, Boult C, Brangman S, et al. Caring for older Americans: the future of geriatric medicine. *J Am Geriatr Soc*. 2005; 53: S245–56.
4. Hughes SL, Weaver FM, Giobbie-Hurder A, et al. Effectiveness of team-managed home-based primary care: a randomized multi-center trial. *JAMA*. 2000; 284: 2877–85.
5. Stuck AE, Egger M, Hammer A, Minder CE, Beck JC. Home visits to prevent nursing home admission and functional decline in elderly people: systematic review and meta-regression analysis. *JAMA*. 2002; 287: 1022–28.
6. Stuck AE, Aronow HU, Steiner A, et al. A trial of annual in-home comprehensive geriatric assessments for elderly people living in the community. *N Engl J Med*. 1995; 333: 1184–89.
7. Centers for Medicare and Medicaid Services. Medicare Physician Fee Schedule Look-Up. Available at: www.cms.hhs.govlphysicians/mpfsapp (accessed 1 November, 2005).
8. Taler G. House calls for the 21st century. *J Am Geriatr Soc*. 1998; 46: 246–48.
9. McWhinney IR. Fourth annual Nicholas J. Pisacano Lecture. The doctor, the patient, and the home: returning to our roots. *J Am Board Fam Pract*. 1997; 10: 430–35.

11

Boy Scouts for Henry

Richard E. Allen, MD, MPH

"MR KORMOS, YOU'RE GOING TO DIE TODAY."

It was his second hospital admission for pneumonia in two months. After nearly 80 years without seeing a doctor, Henry Kormos was again forced by dyspnea to enter my emergency department. He stopped shaking his head and looked up, squinting with one eye and doubting what he'd just heard.

"You're going to die today unless you let me help you," I finished saying. This time there was no mistaking my words. His face twisted in a mix of anger and confusion. He was nearly tied to the bed rails by intravenous lines and nasogastric tubing, and desperately dependent on the large plastic oxygen mask that sustained his labored breathing. His chest was bare and moving rapidly, the ribs forcefully sucking in each breath. Navy tattoos were dark and blurry on his arms, now covered in sweat. A tiny cockroach crawled out of his jeans pocket and onto his belly.

At that moment Mr Kormos wanted nothing more than to kick me, drop all the tubes, and get out of there. I could see in his wrenched face what I had seen before: disgust for modern medicine, but reliance on it for life. I felt unable to share with him my own reservations about interventional medicine. As a second-year resident, I would be laughed to scorn had I recommended comfort measures only.

We had talked through the consent form before. He knew what I needed to do and finally nodded his head once, then dropped his arms and closed his eyes.

The nurse helped me sit him upright, and I performed a thoracentesis to relieve his rapid breathing. Modern medicine triumphed over stubborn Mr Kormos.

The next morning, I introduced him to the medicine team and briefly explained his history. He appeared comfortable now as the crowd of white-coated observers looked in. They debated the merits of computed tomography, bronchoscopy, or both while awaiting cytologic results from the pleural fluid. A chest radiograph showed a fist-sized tumor that filled his right hilum. No doubt the tumor was causing postobstructive pneumonia and would require resection or radiation.

An hour later, I got a call from the nurse. "Your man wants out of here," she said. "He's pulled his IV, and he's stripping his jammies off right now." I ran to the floor.

I was tempted to discharge him with a prescription for oral antibiotics and home oxygen. That option was never mentioned on medicine rounds. No one would suggest giving in to the thing – the cancer or whatever else it was. We are trained instead to fight it at all costs.

I wondered how quickly I could arrange a hospice evaluation, but I had been told they would not come without a pathologically confirmed cancer diagnosis. My cantankerous old friend had no choice but to be subjected to the ways of contemporary hospitalization. He might have stayed home to die, but unfortunately, suffocation is intolerable and brings even the most stubborn of men to beg for our help.

He was struggling to put his pants on as I entered the room. A thin, greasy-haired man stood toward the back. His son, I presumed.

"Mr Kormos, you're very sick," I said, trying to simplify my approach.

"He can't go home," the son said. Henry's son had dumped him on our doorstep to begin with.

"I ain't staying in this place another minute," Mr Kormos said, then paused to hold the mask to his face and force in several breaths.

"Mr Kormos, you have a tumor." I turned to his son, "There's a huge mass in his lungs, and it might be cancer."

"Tumor my eye!" Henry emphatically shook his head.

"Dad, you've got cancer. You've got to stay," emphasized the son. But the words tumor and cancer didn't have the shock effect that I'd hoped for.

Suddenly, Henry collapsed. "Nurse!" I called, catching Henry's fall and pushing him on to the bed. I cranked the oxygen and held the mask tightly to his face. "Let's tube him, and get two new IVs going …" The son stood silently as we worked to save his father's life.

In a week of mechanical ventilation, Mr Kormos continued to fight every needle, scan, and catheter. Hospice care was forgotten as we pushed "a finger or tube in every orifice." Although my name was on the chart, the matter seemed out of my hands as he underwent bronchoscopy, endoscopy, feeding tube insertion, and more. One morning I saw a note with a signature I didn't recognize: "Open biopsy warranted," it read. The new thoracic surgeon in town. "Warranted!" Not "necessary" or "important," but "warranted." And no doubt paid for by Medicare.

It was out of my hands, and Henry's, as the son was convinced by one doctor after another that it was noble to do all these things. To "fight this thing to the bitter end," I could imagine them saying. Like a war with a mortal enemy or a pursuit of a dangerous criminal.

In two months, Henry had improved somewhat and was in stable condition in a nursing home. Modern medicine triumphed once again. One Sunday morning, I took a group of Boy Scouts to visit him. My neighbor said the boys needed a service project, and he asked whether I would take them to visit someone.

Henry was propped up in the bed, naked except for a diaper. I pictured him fighting off the staff as they tried to bathe and clothe him. He looked up to recognize me, like old friends who'd survived the war together. I knew he wouldn't mind the boys coming in, just like medicine rounds in the intensive care unit. They all looked sharp in their tan uniforms. One carried a plate of cookies that my wife had sent along.

"These are my scouts," I spoke loudly for him to hear. He nodded at them, still sucking for air with each inspiration. A portable oxygen machine breathed loudly in the otherwise quiet room. Henry brushed off flies as they landed on his moist skin. He was unkempt, and the room was filthy. I wondered whether he liked it that way or whether the cleaning staff just didn't dare bother old Mr Kormos.

"Can we do anything for you?" I asked. The question was embarrassing. I was embarrassed to be there and to have the boys. I showed them a man who badly needed our charity, but all we had was a plate of cookies. There was cleaning and bathing and feeding to be done. There was probably a home left unoccupied and decrepit. And there was the labor of breathing and the wasting. I felt incapable of offering any real service to him. Only a visit to lessen his loneliness.

Moments passed. "Well, we just wanted to make a visit," I said, to indicate our departure. I paused at the door and let the boys go into the hallway. Then I walked back in alone and sat at the end of Henry's bed.

"I didn't mean to put you through this, Mr Kormos. I wish you could have gone home," I said. Henry looked at me without speaking. He had not spoken in a month. He glared earnestly into my eyes. He blinked frequently and sucked intently on the air mask.

Henry died later that month. I shared the news with my wife and shed a tear of relief. Henry was only the first of several terminally ill patients I have known. To assist their death is criminal, but to prolong a life with no quality may be equally wrong.

Sometimes our patients need help and permission to pass on, a peaceful death uninterrupted by diagnostics and rescue procedures. I think of this when I picture Henry. I daydream of a thin old man, his clean bare chest now breathing comfortably. A smile is on his face. He reminds me that a doctor who cares is the greatest success of modern medicine.

12

Lessons from My Left Foot

Thomas Bodenheimer, MD, MPH

AS A PRIMARY CARE PHYSICIAN, I HAVE CARED FOR PATIENTS WITH chronic illness for decades. I have studied chronic disease. I have tried to improve chronic disease care at several primary care clinics. But it's my left foot that really taught me about chronic disease.

My feet have carried me thousands of miles in my life – walking to work on those hard cement sidewalks, going over high mountain passes with heavy packs. For 25 years I played basketball every Saturday morning on a cement outdoor court, often in old worn-down shoes. Eight months ago, my left foot told me, "Enough abuse. I'm going on strike." Because of the pain, I could bear no weight. I contacted my primary care physician at once. Four medical consultations, two negative imaging studies, and innumerable care plans – immobilization, ice, anti-inflammatories, no weight bearing, taping, wrapping, elevating, and a slew of orthotics – I still could not bear weight on the painful left foot. Diagnosis: soft tissue injury of some sort. Treatment: see what helps and keep doing that. "Maybe you'll be better soon."

It felt chronic. Unable to walk for many weeks without crutches, my life had changed in every way. What did my left foot tell me about how people with chronic conditions feel? The foot taught me four lessons.

First, many people with chronic conditions blame themselves. In my case, it's justified; I have abused my feet. I imagine that the person with diabetes who does not exercise, eats unhealthy foods, and is overweight may also feel a deep self-blame. It is not a helpful feeling even if true. Obsessing about the past and what I could have done to prevent it gets in the way of addressing the future. Perhaps we should be asking patients with chronic conditions whether they blame themselves and help them redirect their thoughts to more productive channels.

Second, I've been blessed with a partner who put her life on hold to take care of me. But I hate to have other people help me. It drags down my sense of self-worth to take and never give. I suspect that many people with functional limitations related to chronic conditions feel the same. Some, of course, have no one to help them. Those who do receive assistance may think themselves worthless, which does not contribute to a therapeutic state of mind.

The third message from my left foot is something that all experts in chronic disease emphasize: depression – the emotional consequence of not being able to do what one is used to. The depression may be worse than the disease. My foot hurts, but my mind hurts 10 times more. Because this depression is a result of the disease, treatment for the depression must include as its major focus a good plan for managing the disease. Also, the depression is variable. When my foot hurts more, my depression deepens. When my foot feels okay, my depression lifts. That is still true eight months later. I remember Professor Kate Lorig, the chronic disease self-management scholar at Stanford, telling me why people with diabetes don't like to do home glucose testing: when they get a high glucose reading, they feel depressed. One sensible response: don't check your glucose levels. Mood can be so variable and so dependent on how a condition is behaving that day – elation with a normal glucose level or blood pressure, a few hours of relief from arthritis pain, some days of freedom from asthma attacks or congestive heart failure exacerbations.

What have I learned beyond what experts have written about chronic conditions and depression? That the depression can be the major aspect of the disease and can pull people down, down, down. That it waxes and wanes along with the disease. And that – adding together the passivity produced by self-blame, the disempowerment fed by needing help from other people, and the "I don't really care what happens" attitude from depression – people with chronic conditions must overcome major challenges to be active participants in their care.

The fourth lesson is about self-efficacy – the feeling of confidence that one can succeed and improve one's life. Self-efficacy is supposed to be activity specific. "I feel 100% sure that I can cook dinner tonight, but I have zero confidence that I can be the winning pitcher in the World Series." Yet an interesting thing happened to me when my left foot revolted and said, "No more walking." Naturally my confidence that I could get from one place to another plummeted. There was also a generalizing effect from that rational loss of confidence. I began to lose my confidence in everything. Can I still write? Can I complete the projects I am committed to doing? Am I a drag to be with? None of these things require my feet, but I began to lose all self-efficacy. The same might happen to others with chronic conditions – losing self-confidence not only for the activities truly limited by the chronic condition, but losing overall confidence in oneself as a human being.

If all these challenges I have experienced are similar to the burdens of the tens of millions of people with chronic conditions, then our obsessive focus on the glycated hemoglobin (HbA1c) levels and peak flow readings may need rethinking. Certainly those outcomes are important, and the four interrelated psychosocial challenges should get better as the glucose levels and peak flow improve. Still, glucose levels and peak flow may not improve until those challenges are discussed and addressed in patients' care plans. I used to think of quality of life or patient experience as second-class measures, not reaching the level of importance held by "hard" clinical outcomes. I failed to consider that a HbA1c level of 8.5% or a low-density cholesterol level of 138 mg/dL is asymptomatic. For many people, pain today trumps a stroke tomorrow. Feeling depressed today obliterates the importance of renal failure tomorrow. Clinical outcomes, such as overall quality of life, percentage of days with pain, or number of depression-free days, may be better patient-centered measures than laboratory numbers.

Eight months after the problem surfaced, I am better but not good. I can walk but not like before. The condition varies from hour to hour, day to day. It has become a chronic problem in partial remission. The anger, self-doubt, and emotional paralysis have gone away. Acceptance has set in. Most importantly, my problem is a musculoskeletal issue about a foot. Not progressive Alzheimer's, not the terrifying dyspnea of congestive heart failure or chronic pulmonary disease. What's the big deal?

Perhaps developing a condition that affected my most cherished activities made me react emotionally to a minor medical condition more than would others with serious disease. Perhaps I'm not as tough as other people. Not everyone with chronic disease becomes depressed and loses self-esteem. I suspect, however, that some of these feelings affect the patients we physicians see but are hidden behind the objective findings that command our attention. In the 15-minute visit, addressing emotions and quality of life simply takes too long.

Did the health care system help me get better? As a physician, I got special treatment. What mattered the most was trust. Since I had no definitive diagnosis, I needed to trust the practitioners trying to help me. Having a trusted family physician and gaining trust in one specialist helped a great deal, even if the only effective treatment turned out to be tincture of time. For the loss of confidence and self-pity, help came from outside the health system: my partner, my coworkers, my friends. Perhaps those of us who provide health care overestimate our own importance and underestimate the critical role of social support – especially when it's lacking.

I'm really mad at my left foot. But I must admit, it has taught me a great deal.

Section 3

Wounds and Healing

It is one of the wonders of human life: each of us experiences wounds, yet we carry the capacity to heal. We begin to heal our lives by changing our relationship with suffering, searching for meaning when we feel most helpless. When we share the suffering of others, we help them to heal as well.[1]

In this section, authors share their stories and ideas about illness, pain, and possibilities for healing.

- *Healing*: what does the concept of "healing" mean for the practice of primary care? Thomas Egnew contends that when physicians focus on curing disease and healing patients' lives, both patient and physician can find wholeness and meaning.
- *Healed*: when he was diagnosed with a life-threatening disease, family physician Roger Rosenblatt received excellent technical care but little compassion. The experience renewed his appreciation for the preciousness of his profession and his life.
- *Touch*: the simple act of touch can soothe and connect us. A clinician's touch, however, is often mediated by the plastic gloves she or he wears to prevent infection. Leif Hass grapples what is lost and gained in the absence of skin-to-skin connection.
- *Courage*: when a patient of 10 years reveals his traumatic life story for the first time, family physician Jon Neher vows to approach conversations with patients with diligence and courage.
- *The Journey*: Patrick Crommett and John Scott – a patient and his family physician – traveled together on a journey of healing. Here, they share the

experience of Patrick's illness and the remarkable relationship that healed them both.

Reference

1. Egnew TR. The meaning of healing: transcending suffering. *Ann Fam Med.* 2005; 3(3): 255–62.

13

Suffering, Meaning, and Healing

Challenges of Contemporary Medicine

Thomas R. Egnew, EdD, LICSW

> *Also, I would like a doctor who is not only a talented physician, but a bit of a metaphysician, too. Someone who can treat body and soul.*
>
> —Anatole Broyard[1(p40)]

DURING 30 YEARS OF TEACHING FAMILY MEDICINE RESIDENTS, I HAVE witnessed many changes in medicine and the image of physicians. As reflected by television, the warm and understanding Dr Marcus Welby (whose program debut was the year family medicine became a specialty) has morphed into the arrogant, cynical Dr Gregory House. Whereas Welby helped patients struggling with transformations in their lives through the strength of his humanity, House condescendingly rescues them from death by sagacity and technology. This evolution seems to mirror changes in medicine grown more technically sophisticated and powerful while physician morale has plummeted and public trust eroded.[2–4] What happened?

Contemporary society has entered a postmodern era in which economic, philosophical, and technological advances have transformed medicine, doctoring, and the doctor-patient relationship.[5] A growing service economy rendered physicians "providers," patients "customers," and medicine a "product." A belief in the relativity of knowledge categorizes biomedicine as but one of a variety of legitimate healing models that vie for patients. The authority of the patient's story of illness now competes with the doctor's story of disease. Doctors are confronted with medical information garnered from the Internet, often of dubious quality and unrelated to the patient's clinical condition. A colleague recently reported having a 9-year-old patient request a hypnotic by brand name, thanks to television advertising. The world of contemporary doctoring has changed!

It seems today's physicians are expected to be an amalgam of Welby's warmth and House's brilliance. As advances in the prevention and treatment of acute disease mean more patients suffer longer with chronic diseases, the traditional medical goals of healing and the relief of suffering become more pressing. Thus, we have entered an era in which the many value questions that arise from and cannot be resolved by a purely curative approach to medicine beg consideration.[6] Saving and prolonging life incur an obligation to accompany patients on their illness journeys, to care for their souls as well as their bodies. Yet, medical training hardly equips physicians to help patients with the metaphysical ramifications of their illnesses.[7]

This essay explores the thesis that contemporary physicians are challenged to both cure disease and to help patients holistically heal, to be physician-healers. It is written with the assumption that a greater appreciation of the nature of holistic healing may help physicians more effectively adapt to a changing world. As social and technical change influence medicine, issues of suffering, meaning, and healing are emerging as integral parts of the work of doctoring. Assuming the role of physician-healer may assist physicians caring for suffering patients, particularly the chronically ill, and may stimulate new meaning to their work.

To illustrate my points, I shall use the words of Anatole Broyard, who chronicled his experience of being doctored while dying of prostate cancer.[1] An author, literary critic, and editor, Broyard astutely observed the human condition and captured his observations in vivid prose. An intellectual, hipster, and Bohemian writer[8] who lived in Greenwich Village during the flowering of the Beat Generation, Broyard powerfully reflects the postmodern mentality that influences contemporary doctoring.

Suffering, Meaning, & Healing

Holistic healing may be understood as "the personal experience of the transcendence of suffering."[9] Suffering is an intrinsically disagreeable experience that is angst of an order different from pain, though it may involve pain.[10] It arises from

perceptions of impending destruction of an individual's personhood and continues until the threat of disintegration has passed or the integrity of the person
is restored in some other manner.[11] As such, suffering subsumes nonphysical
dimensions – social, psychological, cultural, spiritual – associated with being a
person that are relatively unaddressed in medical training.[9,11,12]

Suffering is personal, individual, and commonly expressed as a narrative.[13,14]
"My initial experience of illness was as a series of disconnected shocks," Broyard
reported, "and my first instinct was to try to bring it under control by turning
it into a narrative. Always in emergencies we invent narratives."[1(p19)] Although
sources of suffering may be shared in common – e.g., the massive loss of life
caused by the 2004 Indian Ocean tsunami – the particulars of suffering for any
individual remain exclusively personal and anecdotal. The conventional expectation of narrative involving a past leading into a present that foretells a foreseeable
future is "wrecked" by illness.[15] The present is not what the past was supposed
to foreshadow, and the future is too frightening to contemplate.

Because suffering arises from the meaning ascribed to events, it engenders a
crisis of meaning[16] as previous meanings attributed to the sufferer's experience no
longer apply.[17] The patient's suffering must be heard and accepted, as the denial
of the patient's story of suffering and sacrifice is a denial of the patient's identity
as a sufferer.[18] "To the typical physician, my illness is a routine incident in his
rounds," Broyard observed, "while for me it's the crisis of my life. I would feel better if I had a doctor who at least perceived this incongruity."[1(p43)] Suffering fills the
chasm of meaninglessness that opens when the patient's previously held meaning
structures have been destroyed and new ones are yet to be constructed.[17] The
physician-healer affirms the sense of meaninglessness conveyed in the patient's
narrative and then helps the patient to create or discover a healing narrative with
new meanings that transcend suffering.[19]

Transcending Suffering

Suffering may be resolved if the threat to integrity is removed, distress relieved,
and integrity of personhood reconstituted to resume purposeful engagement
with the world. Not all suffering can be resolved, and some types are beyond
medicine.[20,21] Still, suffering can be transcended through acceptance, through
the creation of new connections with the world, and through finding meaning in
the experience of suffering.

Transcendence means "extending or lying beyond the limits of ordinary experience."[22] It reflects a change in the patient's relationships to the illness,[23] to others, and to the world that results in rising above the suffering previously experienced. It entails flowing with or adapting to changes from the patient's ordinary experience induced by life cycle events, disease, trauma, or degeneration. Transcendence is categorically different from being cured of disease, and cure does not equate to healing. Transcendence of suffering through holistic healing can occur regardless of cure, restoration of health, continued illness or impairment, or impending death.[9]

How does acceptance help patients transcend suffering? Intactness of personhood is forged through attachments to those aspects by which one identifies oneself as a person and defines one's sense of meaning and purpose in life. The severing of an attachment precipitates suffering as it disrupts the previous sense of personal integrity with its attendant senses of meaning.[13,24] By accepting the change and neither pursuing nor rejecting the severed attachment, suffering is transcended.[25,26]

Acceptance can be assisted by normalizing the patient's feelings and responses to illness. "It is only natural for a patient to feel some disgust at the change brought about in his body by illness," Broyard observed, "and I wonder whether an innovative doctor couldn't find a way to reconceptualize this situation."[1(p48)] The physician-healer helps the patient discover opportunities for growth in the most dire of circumstances, and the ability to transcend suffering exists even in the presence of the most frightening of diseases. For example, a substantial percentage of advanced cancer patients report little or no suffering,[27] and there is ample witness to the peace evinced by persons who have accepted their impending deaths.[28,29]

For the suffering patient, acceptance often results in a personal style for handling the illness, as Broyard described: "... every seriously ill person needs to develop a style for his illness. I think that only by insisting on your style can you keep from falling out of love with yourself as the illness attempts to diminish or disfigure you."[1(p25)] This style reflects a new sense of identity. "You don't really know that you're ill until the doctor tells you so. When he tells you you're ill," wrote Broyard, "this is not the same as giving you permission to be ill. You eke out your illness. You'll always be an amateur in your illness."[1(p37)] A new sense of integrity, a new connection to the world and to others, a new way of being emerges.

Suffering is also transcended by investiture with meaning. Because suffering arises in a void of meaninglessness, discovering meaning transforms the experience. "Suffering ceases to be suffering in some way," Victor Frankl observed, "at the moment it finds a meaning."[30] Thus, the extremely ill Pope John Paul II, unable to perform his Pontifical duties during Holy Week, announced he was "uniting his sufferings with those of Christ"[31] and invested his illness experience with a meaning that transcended his suffering. "Meaning," physician Jeff Kane has argued, "is as central to healing as the skeleton is to the body."[23] Broyard concurred: "Any meaning of illness is better than none."[1(p65)]

Healing Connections

Sickness separates persons from wholeness with the world as known in health. "My friends flatter me by calling my performance courageous or gallant," wrote Broyard, "but my doctor should know better. He should be able to imagine the aloneness of the critically ill, a solitude as haunting as a Chirico painting."[1(p42)] To ameliorate isolation, the physician-healer becomes a "therapeutic instrument," providing relationships to "reconnect sick persons to the world of the well."[32] Toward this end, continuity of caring relationships through time and the patient's feeling of being known are very important aspects of healing.[9,33]

Therapeutic contact involves a therapeutic alliance facilitated by empathy, warmth, and genuineness.[34] Being "heard and accepted" goes beyond an intellectual understanding of the sufferer's plight. It entails the development of a relationship that links the patient, at a minimum through the doctor-patient relationship, to a community that turns toward a new future despite the changes the patient has experienced.

Suchman and Matthews described the therapeutic relationship as having a "connexional," transpersonal dimension that bonds physician and patient in "a sensation of wholeness.[35] "I wouldn't demand a lot of my doctor's time: I just wish he would brood on my situation for perhaps five minutes," Broyard proclaimed, "that he would give me his whole mind just once, be bonded with me for a brief space, survey my soul as well as my flesh, to get at my illness, for each man is ill in his own way."[1(p44)] In connexion, both physician and patient are vulnerable to the risks intrinsic to transpersonal intimacy.[33,36] "The sick man asks far too much," wrote Broyard, "he is impatient with everything, and his doctor may be afraid of making a fool of himself in trying to reply."[1(p54)] Yet, sharing vulnerability opens the possibility of a healing connection around the commonality of human woundedness.[37]

The compassion that fosters a therapeutic alliance and enhances knowledge of another's suffering is aided by empathy,[38] which requires a willingness to suffer some of the patient's pain in the sharing of suffering that is vital to healing.[33,37,39,40]

The empathic understanding that ensues from a strong therapeutic alliance allows physician-healers to actively and intentionally guide patients in rewriting their life narratives to affirm normalcy, establish acceptance, discover meaning, make new connections to the world, transcend suffering, and experience healing.[9,36,41]

Because healing is a process,[42] the metamorphosis of the role of doctor to healer is the change from doer to helper,[43] from expert problem solver and fixer to servant and companion, an accompanier on the healing journey.

Healing and Narrative

The work of healing is often a work of narration, of eliciting the patient's illness story and then helping the patient discover a new, healing story.[19] "Stories," claimed Broyard, "are antibodies against illness and pain."[1(p20)] This narrative work requires understanding the format of illness stories and knowing how to help patients edit their stories. Illness stories reflect descriptions of experiences of devastation, reflection, and response. They portray broad truths of the patient's experience of illness and life, are interpretable and invested with an emotional core, and must be told in the style of the teller.[23]

The physician-healer creates a safe environment for patients to reveal their stories by encouraging storytelling.[19] Toward this end, physicians must belay intentions to heal, and suspend personal views and values so they can enter the patient's world without bias.[23,44] What the sick man wants most from people, according to Broyard, "is not love but an appreciative critical grasp of his situation, what is known now in the literature of illness as 'empathetic witnessing.' The patient is always on the brink of revelation, and he needs an amanuensis."[1(p44)] An amanuensis is an individual who can skillfully transcribe speech!

How are healing narratives developed? Ultimately, this work is the patient's, for it is the patient's healing. To help, physician-healers must be competent in narrative medicine.[19,45] They must ground the medical story in the patient's experience,[46] which necessitates a patient-centered approach,[47] and they must be curious about their patients' stories. Curiosity is best expressed through circular questions that directly address the patient's concerns and invite embellishment of the story.[19] "Besides talking himself," Broyard observed, "the doctor ought to bleed the patient of talk, of the consciousness of his illness, as earlier physicians used to bleed their patients to let out heat or dangerous humors."[1(p53)]

Physician-healers also help patients cope with the impersonality of technology by connecting the patient's illness narrative with the technomedical story.

"Since technology deprives me of the intimacy of my illness, makes it not mine but something that belongs to science," observed Broyard, "I wish my doctor could somehow repersonalize it for me."[1(p47)] Helping patients to make this connection, Broyard maintained, allows patients to better own their illnesses. The disease story must be connected with the illness narrative for a patient to create a healing narrative, a style for living with the illness.[46]

By drawing out the patient's experience, the connections made in ascribing meaning to their illnesses, physician-healers help patients move through the processes of devastation to reflection and on to a new narrative that increases the ability to respond to the changes wrought by the illness. All aspects of the medical encounter can be used to help patients towards healing.[48] Consider the patient who, after years of progressive debilitation with negative workups, wept with joy when finally diagnosed with multiple sclerosis. "Now I know I'm not crazy," the patient cried. "Whether he wants to be or not, the doctor is a story-teller," maintained Broyard, "and he can turn our lives into good or bad stories, regardless of the diagnosis."[1(p53)]

Back to the Future

As medicine evolves in the postmodern era, the clinical skills needed to manage a growing population of chronically ill patients will become increasingly important. An acute care, subspecialty, curative model of service delivery is insufficient for the needs of the chronically ill.[49] Healing requires continuity of relationships to nurture the intimacy that permits the exploration of the meaning of illness.[9,33] Toward this end, the Future of Family Medicine's call for a "medical home" with "patient-centered care," and a "whole-person orientation"[50] is very appropriate – but only viable if staffed by physician-healers skilled in helping patients transcend suffering.

The physician-healer must know how to actively diagnose suffering and explore its origins if detected. Doing so involves (1) direct questioning, (2) appreciating the sounds and sights of suffering, (3) sensing the loss of connection with patients who have withdrawn into their suffering, and (4) empathic identification.[38] The diagnosis of suffering is uniquely dependent upon the clinician's subjective experience, making physician-healers "strange instruments."[51]

To manage the shared vulnerability of the close interpersonal relationships of healing, physician-healers must be mindful so they can balance their personal responses to patients with their professional presentation.[52] Not allowing their own feelings and views to cloud a clear appreciation of the patient's experience permits physician-healers to affirmatively witness the patient's suffering.[53] By cultivating such personal insight, physicians can manage any countertransference that is potentially harmful to the healing milieu.[54]

The change from expert-doer to servant-accompanier requires that physicians attend to how they are with patients as much as what they do for them.[48] Empathic connection is not simply a nice relational attribute; it has physiologic impacts.[55] The chronically ill and their families need remoralization,[56] making the physician-healer a morale catalyst. Physician-healers both cure disease and heal the sick. They use science to treat disease but draw on themselves to explore the meaning patients append to their illness experience and to guide healing. As evidence-based medicine guru David Sackett observed: "The most powerful therapeutic tool you'll ever have is your own personality."[57]

Whether physicians can be healers in a postmodern era in which medicine is an industry with clinic volumes that curtail meaningful dialogue with patients is a concern.[33,42,58] This is perhaps the greatest challenge for contemporary medicine and the central struggle for its soul: Is the heart of medicine to be centered upon holistic healing or upon the adept dispersal of biomedical services as a market commodity? A health care delivery system focused on holistic healing would undoubtedly be tooled differently than our current model. At a minimum, it would promote access to and continuity of care, provide for home visits, equitably reimburse spending time with (rather than doing things to) patients, and provide parity in funding for mental health issues.

Skeptics will note that nothing written here is new. This is true. Whether it is Hippocrates' hypothesis, "It is more important to know what sort of person has a disease than to know what sort of disease a person has"[59]; or Osler's admonition, "Care more particularly for the individual patient than for the special features of the disease"[60]; or Peabody's opinion, "The secret of the care of the patient is caring for the patient"[61]; or Remen's reflection, "The practice of medicine is a special kind of love,"[62] the principle is the same: healing is stimulated through the medium of close, caring interpersonal relationships. So it has been; so it shall be.

Once, physicians had little to offer patients except the strength of their personalities. With the advent of biomedicine, personality gave way to science and technology. The success of biomedicine requires contemporary physicians to connect personally with patients to heal the illnesses their technology can so forcefully sustain. "Just as a mother ushers her child into the world," Broyard proclaimed, "so the doctor must usher the patient out of the world of the healthy and into whatever physical and mental purgatory awaits him. The doctor is the patient's only familiar in a foreign country."[1(p55)] To not accompany patients on their illness journeys is to abandon them in a foreign world of sickness.

Some physicians may feel overwhelmed by the idea of assuming a healer role when time and energy are already at a premium. But not every patient coming to the physician needs healing. Most will not be suffering, nor will all who suffer need healing. Many will heal spontaneously as the miracles of cure remove any threat to the patient and allow reconnection with life as previously known. But all patients will eventually fail, and medicine's power to prolong suffering is immense, so all patients will eventually need a skilled physician-healer.

Finally, developing the role of physician-healer may not only better serve the chronically ill but may also stem the tide of physician burnout and restore a sense of awe and mystery to medicine by reinstating the personal power of the physician as a therapeutic agent.[33] As Broyard surmised: "Not every patient can be saved, but his illness may be eased by the way the doctor responds to him – and in responding to him the doctor may save himself …. In learning to talk to his patients, the doctor may talk himself back into loving his work. He has little to lose and everything to gain by letting the sick man into his heart."[1(p57)]

References

1. Broyard A. *Intoxicated by My Illness*. New York, NY: Fawcett Columbine; 1992.
2. Steiger B. Survey results: doctors say morale is hurting. *Physician Exec*. 2006; 32(6): 6–15.
3. Crawshaw R. Diminished medical morale syndrome. A profession's impairment. *J S C MedAssoc*. 2000; 96(7): 304–09.
4. Mechanic D. Changing medical organization and the erosion of trust. *Milbank Q*. 1996; 74(2): 171–89.
5. Morris DB. How to speak postmodern. Medicine, illness, and cultural change. *Hastings Cent Rep*. 2000; 30(6): 7–16.
6. Veatch RM. Contemporary bioethics and the demise of modern medicine. In: Ormiston G, Sassower R, eds. *Prescriptions: The Dissemination of Medical Authority*. New York, NY: Greenwood Press; 1990: 22–39.
7. Rich BA. Postmodern medicine: deconstructing the Hippocratic Oath. *Forum Appl Res Public Policy*. 1993; 65(1): 77–136.
8. Mitgang H. Anatole Broyard, 70, book critic and editor at the Times, is dead. *New York Times*. 1990 Oct 12; Sect. A: 26 (col 1–3).
9. Egnew TR. The meaning of healing: transcending suffering. *Ann Fam Med*. 2005; 3(3): 255–62.
10. Chapman CR, Gavrin J. Suffering and its relationship to pain. *J Palliat Care*. 1993; 9(2): 5–13.
11. Cassell EJ. The nature of suffering and the goals of medicine. *N Engl J Med*. 1982; 306(11): 639–45.
12. Cassell EJ. The nature of suffering: physical, psychological, social, and spiritual aspects. In Starck PL, McGovern JP, eds. *The Hidden Dimension of Illness: Human Suffering*. New York, NY: NLN Publications; 1992. pp. 1–10.

13. Moerman DE. Physiology and symbols: the anthropological implications of the placebo effect. In: Romanucci-Ross L, Moerman D, Tancredi L, eds. *The Anthropology of Medicine: From Culture to Method*. South Hadley, MA: J. F. Bergin Publishers; 1983: 156–67.

14. Reich WT. Speaking of suffering: a moral account of compassion. *Soundings*. 1989; 72(1): 83–108.

15. Frank AW. *The Wounded Storyteller*. Chicago, IL: University of Chicago Press; 1995.

16. Barrett DA. Suffering and the process of transformation. *J Pastoral Care*. 1999; 53(4): 461–72.

17. Kahn DL, Steeves RH. An understanding of suffering grounded in clinical practice and research. In Ferrell BR, ed. *Suffering*. Sudbury, MA: Jones and Bartlett Publishers; 1996: 3–27.

18. Amato JA. *Victims and Values: A History and a Theory of Suffering*. New York, NY: Praeger Publishers; 1990.

19. Launer J. *Narrative-Based Primary Care: A Practical Guide*. Oxford: Radcliffe Medical Press; 2002.

20. Buddhism. In: Hitchcock ST, Esposito JL, Tutu D, Tutu M, eds. *Geography of Religion: Where God Lives, Where Pilgrims Walk*. Washington, DC: National Geographic Society; 2004. pp. 132–97.

21. Fleischer TE. Suffering reclaimed: medicine according to Job. *Perspect Biol Med*. 1999; 42(4): 475–88.

22. *Webster's New Collegiate Dictionary*. Springfield MA: G & C Merriam Company; 1979. p. 1230.

23. Kane J. *How to Heal: A Guide for Caregivers*. New York, NY: Helios Press; 2003.

24. Kegan R. *The Evolving Self*. Cambridge, MA; Harvard University Press; 1982.

25. Mikulas WL. Four noble truths of Buddhism related to behavior therapy. *Psychol Rec*. 1978; 28: 59–67.

26. Hayes SC, Smith S. *Get Out of Your Mind and Into Your Life: The New Acceptance and Commitment Therapy*. Oakland, CA: New Harbinger Publications; 2005.

27. Wilson KG, Chochinov HM, McPherson CJ, et al. Suffering with advanced cancer. *J Clin Oncol*. 2007; 25(13): 1691–97.

28. Albom M. *Tuesdays With Morrie: An Old Man, A Young Man, and Life's Greatest Lessons*. New York, NY: Doubleday; 1997.

29. Buchwald A. *Too Soon to Say Goodbye*. New York, NY: Random House; 2006.

30. Frankl VE. *Man's Search for Meaning: An Introduction to Logotherapy*. New York, NY: Pocket Books; 1984.

31. Pope says he's uniting his pain with Christ's, will miss services. *The News Tribune*. 2005; March 19; Sect. A:3(col. 1).

32. Cassell EJ. *The Nature of Suffering and the Goals of Medicine*. New York, NY: Oxford University Press; 1991.

33. Scott JG, Cohen D, DiCicco-Bloom B, Miller WL, Stange KC, Crabtree BF. Understanding healing relationships in primary care. *Ann Fam Med*. 2008; 6(4): 315–22.

34. Hubble MA, Duncan BL, Miller SC. *The Heart & Soul of Change: What Works in Therapy*. Washington DC. American Psychological Association; 1999.

35. Suchman AL, Matthews DA. What makes the patient-doctor relationship therapeutic? Exploring the connexional dimension of medical care. *Ann Intern Med*. 1988; 108(1): 125–30.

36. Matthews DA, Suchman AL, Branch LT Jr. Making "connexions": enhancing the therapeutic potential of patient-clinician relationships. *Ann Intern Med*. 1993; 118(12): 973–77.

37. Nouwen HJM. *The Wounded Healer*. New York, NY: Image Books; 1979.

38. Cassell EJ. Recognizing suffering. *Hastings Cent Rep*. 1991; 21(3): 24–31.

39. Pellegrino ED. The healing relationship: the architectonics of clinical medicine. In: Shelp EA, ed. *The Clinical Encounter: The Moral Fabric of the Physician-Patient Relationship*. Dordrecht, Holland: D. Reidel Publishing; 1983. pp. 153–72.

40. Jackson SW. The listening healer in the history of psychological healing. *Am J Psychiatry*. 1992; 149(12): 1623–32.

41. Farber SJ, Egnew TR, Herman-Bertsch JL. Defining effective clinician roles in end-of-life care. *J Fam Pract*. 2002; 51(2): 153–58.

42. Hsu C, Phillips WR, Sherman KJ, Hawkes R, Cherkin DC. Healing in primary care: a vision shared by patients, physicians, nurses, and clinical staff. *Ann Fam Med*. 2008; 6(4): 307–14.

43. Hammerschlag CA. *The Theft of the Spirit: A Journey to Spiritual Healing With Native Americans*. New York, NY: Simon & Schuster; 1993.

44. Rogers CR. *A Way of Being*. Boston, MA: Houghton Mifflin Company; 1980.

45. Charon R. *Narrative Medicine: Honoring the Stories of Illness*. New York, NY: Oxford University Press; 2006.

46. Hunter KM. *Doctor's Stories*. Princeton, NJ: Princeton University Press; 1991.

47. Stewart M, Brown JB, Weston WW, McWhinney IR, Freeman TR. *Patient-Centered Medicine. Transforming the Clinical Method*. Thousand Oaks, CA: Sage Publications; 1995.

48. Adler HM. The history of the present illness as treatment: who's listening, and why does it matter? *J Am Board Fam Pract*. 1997; 10(1): 28–35.

49. Fox E. Predominance of the curative model of medical care. A residual problem. *JAMA*. 1997; 278(9): 761–63.

50. Martin JC, Avant RF, Bowman MA, et al. The future of family medicine: a collaborative project of the family medicine community. *Ann Fam Med*. 2004; 2(Suppl 1): S3–S32.

51. Cassell EJ. Diagnosing suffering: a perspective. *Ann Intern Med*. 1999; 131(7): 531–34.

52. Epstein RM. Mindful practice. *JAMA*. 1999; 282(9): 833–39.

53. Dass R, Gorman P. *How Can I Help?* New York, NY: Alfred A Knopf; 1991.

54. Marshall AA, Smith RC. Physicians' emotional reactions to patients: recognizing and managing countertransference. *Am J Gastroenterol*. 1995; 90(1): 4–8.

55. Adler HM. The sociophysiology of caring in the doctor-patient relationship. *J Gen Intern Med*. 2002; 17(11): 883–90.

56. Kleinman A. *The Illness Narratives*. New York, NY: Basic Books; 1988.

57. Smith R. Thoughts for new medical students at a new medical school. *BMJ*. 2003; 327(7429): 1430–33.

58. Rastegar DA. Health care becomes an industry. *Ann Fam Med*. 2004; 2(1): 79–83.

59. Xplore, Inc. [Web site]. www.brainyquote.com/quotes/authors/h/hippocrates.html (accessed Jul 8, 2008).

60. Silverman ME, Murray TJ, Brayan CS, eds. *The Quotable Osler*. Philadelphia, PA: American College of Physicians; 2003.

61. Peabody FW. The care of the patient. *JAMA*. 1927; 88: 877–82.

62. Remen NR. *Kitchen Table Wisdom*. New York, NY: Riverhead Books; 2006.

14

Getting the News

Roger A. Rosenblatt, MD, MPH, MFR

"COME TAKE A LOOK AT THIS," THE PATHOLOGIST SAID. HE AND THE urologist were peering through the separate eyepieces of a teaching microscope. I looked at the specimen, stained a delicate pink and blue, and followed as he showed me the nests of cancer cells infiltrating the normal architecture of the surrounding prostate gland. As I looked at the spread of these malignant interlopers, I felt dizzy.

"You guys go on without me," I said. "I'll meet you back in the room." The "room" was a gloomy examining room in the nearby urology clinic, adorned with pictures of diseased prostates. So I went and sat, still a bit unsteady, on the examining table. The prostate tissue was mine, the brightly colored product of a biopsy done two weeks earlier.

My colleagues at University Hospital assumed that I would want to join them in reviewing the biopsy. The biopsy was critical in selecting the best treatment option; the virulence, extent, and distribution of the cancer would determine whether I had a chance of being cured. But their fascinating intellectual exercise was my potential death sentence. Perhaps they thought that I would be comforted by assuming the mantle of physician as I looked at these crisp slices of myself under the lens. Being a physician did not inoculate me from the terror of confronting the reality that I had cancer.

I had gotten the first inkling of the biopsy results the week earlier in the disembodied text of an e-mail, sent by the urologist's assistant. The e-mail read: "Have you looked at the path report yet? Call the urology clinic and make an immediate appointment." While not exactly informative, it was clear that the news wasn't good. The biopsy had been excruciating, but this was worse. After being skewered like a shish kebab, the e-mail was like a second biopsy needle, but this time through the heart. Furthermore, I was expected to review the pathology results by myself, using our university's electronic medical record.

Looking at the pathology report on the computer was a devastating experience. The first reading of the biopsy did not look promising: the cells were quite malignant, and there were lots of them spread liberally throughout my hapless prostate gland. By pure chance my family physician had come to the university for a medical conference, and I waited until he stopped by my office to actually look at the report. Having a caring human being with me helped me deal with the shock, though it still seemed like a terrible way to convey the information.

The subsequent staging of my cancer was a cascade of successive tortures. Blood draws rarely succeeded on the first try, and by the time I made it to surgery, most of my veins had collapsed in protest. The interminable CAT scan occurred in the evening, long after the radiologists had gone home, meaning that I got to sweat out the results through the ensuing sleepless night. Colleagues whom I had not told of my disease came up and commiserated: I appreciated their concern, but it was clear that medical privacy was unlikely in an institution where I had worked for 30 years. In fact, as I went through the diagnostic mill, treating physicians would tell me stories about the cancers of others on the staff, thinking it would make me feel better to know that I wasn't alone. Although it had that effect, I also realized that my case would be grist for future discussions among my colleagues.

By the time I made it to the surgical suite, I was a wreck. The surgery went well – the surgeon was talented, quick, and detached – and the final prognosis was better than the biopsy had suggested. The experience, however, was very traumatic, and not only because of the life-threatening nature of the underlying illness.

Does it have to be this way? Perhaps it does. The very things that make tertiary centers what they are – high patient volumes, complex technology, and efficiency – also make it difficult to forge nurturing relationships between healers and patients. Skilled specialists taking care of critically ill patients need to distance themselves to maintain their own emotional equilibrium. I made the task more difficult for my physicians because I was so much like them, and I understand why they treated me more like a physician than a patient. Family physicians can mitigate, but not annul, the terrors of serious disease, and they live in the same shadow of mortality that falls on everyone.

The lessons I learned from this journey reverberate through my personal and professional life. My medical students and patients helped me regain my footing, and I realize what a precious gift it is to be able to help other people realize their

The Wonder and the Mystery

own dreams. I spend more time with my family and no longer form judgments or give advice. And I listen – to the wind, the birds, and to my fellow creatures who wrestle with the mystery, majesty, and pain of their own brief sojourn on earth.

15

Losing Touch in the Era of Superbugs?

Leif Hass, MD

THE PLASTIC GLOVES I PUT ON AS I ENTER THE PATIENT'S ROOM ARE TWO sizes too small. They pull at the hairs on the back of my hand. Locating them, putting them on, disposing of them, all add to the sense of busyness that pervades my days as a hospitalist. Then, of course, there is the physical separation that the gloves create – something that gives me pause.

The room I enter is that of Mr Jones, a 54-year-old man with poorly controlled diabetes and a 1-cm ulcer on his left great toe. I explain, in what has become an extended part of my introduction of myself, that I wear gloves when I examine all patients to curb the spread of germs. As is typical, I hear no hint of disappointment from him, but for me, there inevitably is a slight sense of loss as I proceed with my examination.

Mr Jones leads a life that appears to have little intimacy. He lives alone in a notoriously rundown residential hotel where he keeps to himself to avoid the violence that plagues his neighborhood. Upon admission, he detailed to me with frustration the difficulties he has had getting care. Last week when he called a county clinic about his blood glucose levels of 350 mg/dL, he was told to follow-up in four weeks. Getting Mr Jones's glucose levels down and treating his foot infection won't be enormously difficult, but in the long run what he needs to improve his health is to feel invested in his relationship with the health care system. Faith in one doctor might provide him with the perseverance he needs to connect with another doctor in the haphazard world of safety-net health care. Any distancing could jeopardize the building of trust essential in a good doctor-patient relationship. I am afraid he might experience my use of gloves as a desire to keep an emotional in addition to a physical distance.

Leaving Mr Jones's room, I hear cries in Cantonese from another patient of mine, Ms Chua. She is 89 years old with advanced dementia, and she had been sent from the nursing home because of increasing agitation and a fever. Twenty-four hours into her admission her fever has abated, but she has remained agitated. I enter the room, speak in soothing tones, and gently stroke her forehead. The smooth glide of skin on skin is missing. My hands, sweaty in the vinyl gloves, move less fluidly than they otherwise would. There is a loss of what could have been a brief soothing moment for us both. Even in her delirium, I imagine she can tell this is an institutional comforting because of the feel and smell of plastic.

My sense of loss commingles with ongoing ruminations about the consequences of not having started to wear gloves sooner. I have always thought I was a good hand-washer, but if I had been wearing gloves routinely last year, perhaps my daughter and I would not have been hospitalized with methicillin-resistant *Staphylococcus aureus* (MRSA).

Last year Josephine, my 10-year-old daughter, scraped her knee on the playground; for two weeks it was sore, and then suddenly it was red and warm. I started her on trimethoprim-sulfamethoxazole; even so, she had a temperature of 102 degrees the next day, so we brought her to the hospital, where she stayed for three days getting antibiotics.

A month after that, I developed pain in my arm without any redness or swelling. In an effort not to doctor myself, I saw an orthopedist who thought it was a biceps tear and put me in a splint. Two days later, I returned from work in worse pain and exhausted. After I collapsed on the couch, Josephine took off my splint and made the diagnosis. "Daddy," she said, "you have the same infection I had. You need to go to the hospital."

I had developed a deep tissue infection without a clear port of entry and, as were my daughter's, my wound cultures were positive for MRSA. During my hospitalization I was happy to be handled with gloved hands. I needed a couple of surgeries to ensure the wound was clean then went home on intravenous vancomycin.

My wife, an epidemiologist, asked about treating our other young children and sterilizing the environment after our daughter's hospitalization. I explained that, despite my urge to treat the whole family with mupirocin and topical antibacterial soap, I was following the recommendations of the pediatric infectious disease guy I had cornered during my daughter's hospital stay. "MRSA is pandemic," he said. "There is no reason to treat it differently than other skin infections."

When I was hospitalized, my wife, at home with our three young children, was immediately on the telephone with her physician colleagues and getting informal consultations from national authorities on staphylococcus. She also got a good dose of MRSA horror stories – including tales of loss of limbs, life, and recurrent infections in colonized households. When I got home, she and the kids were on a 2-drug regimen and getting daily chlorhexidine baths. Never was a house so clean, but with an invisible threat, it remained hard to feel entirely safe.

My return to work after my illness was more difficult than I like to admit. I reflected on my training in family medicine at San Francisco General Hospital. I learned to focus on the whole patient rather than their specific ailments. Sometimes 50% of patients in my care had human immunodeficiency virus (HIV). Advanced HIV brought with it other infectious concerns, such as tuberculosis, but I went about my work fearlessly out of professional duty and solidarity with my patients. I remember feeling self-righteous at what I believed were overly vigilant and stigmatizing precautions being taken by other health professionals. I hoped these memories would bolster my determination to "lay on the hands" again. But the hospital wards that had been so familiar now seemed like uncontrollable pools of pathogens the rest of the staff managed to blithely ignore. In every patient I saw threats to my family and myself. In addition to wearing gloves and now a white coat as well, I washed my hands, stethoscope, pagers, and pens obsessively. This behavior has improved with time, but I still feel that I am putting my family at risk every day I go to work. Given the trajectory of drug resistance, it is hard to imagine these thoughts will ever entirely go away – nor do I honestly think they should.

I understand objectively that I do not need to wear gloves with all my patients, but for a great number of patients, all clinicians must take considerable precautions to prevent the spread of infection. Guidelines support the use of alcohol-based foam products rather than gloves except when multidrug-resistant pathogens are confirmed, but given the increasing rates and virulence of these organisms, I am not convinced such measures will continue to be enough to protect our patients.[1,2] I know, however, another important reason I now wear gloves is out of fear for my family and me.

Yet I see touch as a communication tool. For me, touch is particularly important when trying to bridge large socioeconomic and cultural gaps. A hand on the shoulder or the knee or a thoughtful physical examination, I believe, can make a patient understand at a deep nonverbal level you are there for them. I work hard to demonstrate concern for my patients with tone of voice, facial expressions, and body language, yet I feel I am losing some connectedness without skin-to-skin contact.

At the end of the day I go back to see Mr Jones to relay to him some good news. His bone scan suggests he does not have osteomyelitis. With the news of his scan, Mr Jones smiles for the first time in the three days I've been seeing him. "I guess I'll be getting out of here in a couple of days then. You'll follow me in your office, won't ya doc?"

I put a gloved hand on his shoulder and say "I don't see patients outside of the hospital, but I'll send you to see my buddy at the downtown clinic; she'll do you right."

"That's what I need, doc. Someone I can count on."

"You're a good man, Mr Jones," I say as I prepare to leave the room. "It's going to take hard work to get yourself healthy again, but I know you can do it."

As I toss my gloves in the trash and head out of the room, I realize that the people most in need of touch – those who have the greatest need to connect with a fellow human being, those I did not hesitate to touch without gloves in the past – have now become those I am most hesitant to touch without them. I am working up to not wearing gloves all the time. I hope that as I do become more relaxed, I won't stop paying attention to nonverbal communication or the psychological consequences of illness, and my patients don't end up feeling dehumanized by their hospitalization. We must not "lose touch" with what it is to provide patient-centered care as we navigate the increasingly complicated world of medicine in the 21st century.

References

1. Siegel JD, Rhinehart E, Jackson M, Chiarello L, the Healthcare Infection Control Practices Advisory Committee. *Management of Multidrug-resistant Organisms in Healthcare Setting.* Washington, DC: Centers for Disease Control; 2006.
2. Hand hygiene in healthcare settings. Centers for Disease Control and Prevention Web site. www.cdc.gov/HandHygiene/index.html (accessed Mar 3, 2009). Updated May 5, 2010.

16

The Decade Dance

Jon O. Neher, MD

MR. KELLEY (NOT HIS REAL NAME) SITS ON THE EXAMINATION TABLE, A collection of tics and spasms, refusing to meet my gaze. His obvious anxiety suggests that he is building up to some important disclosure. "You know," he finally says, looking out the window, "I've never told anybody about this. ..." He clears his throat. "I was sexually abused as a kid."

I stare at him blankly a moment, his statement not registering. Then slowly, the enormity of what he just said starts to sink in. "I'm sorry to hear that," I tell him, knowing the words are inadequate. His revelation, however, instantly sheds a chilling light on his many and chronic peculiarities.

Ten years ago, I had welcomed him into my practice and took my first history and performed my first physical examination on him. At the time, he was in his early forties, with thinning red hair but a boyish, freckled face. Throughout his initial visit (and ever since), he avoided making eye contact and spoke only in short, nervous sentences. I noted in the chart that he had never married, and he reported no close friends. Although I was concerned about his social isolation, he seemed so acutely ill at ease that I thought it might actually be unkind to press for more details. I promised myself I would ask about it later, but never did.

Eight years ago, I found a small melanoma on his back. Mr. Kelley had accepted the news as if it was of no consequence, as if the possibility of disfigurement or death was a mere annoyance. Fortunately, he did well medically. Mr. Kelley, I now understood, had already faced far greater challenges than skin cancer.

Four years ago, Mr. Kelley developed a rectal prolapse that required surgical repair. I asked him if he had any thoughts about why the condition might have developed. Mr. Kelley said only that he had a problem with chronic constipation.

That explanation seemed to be enough for the surgeon. I don't think the surgeon or I even considered the possibility of perineal injury.

Back in the present, Mr. Kelley tugs at his collar and coughs. "I was fired from my job, too."

"When was that?" I ask.

"Last week."

Two years ago, Mr. Kelley had been injured at his job in a warehouse when he slipped on a wet floor and hurt his back. Although lumbar imaging showed only some arthritis and minor disk disease, his pain incapacitated him. The episode also unleashed from him a torrent of anger. As I filled out innumerable work capacity forms, white-hot rage poured out of him at my office. It poured out of him at the job site too, until everyone there became just a little afraid of him, marking him as the type of man who might just "go postal."

Part of his anger was directed at his injury and his work situation. But I knew the man well enough by now to suspect that, at its root, this rage went far deeper. I suggested that he see a counselor for anger management. Initially reluctant, he eventually followed through on the suggestion. Those anger management sessions must have been effective. He now knew with absolute certainty where his anger was coming from.

"The abuse went on for years, you know," he adds. A sardonic grin flashes across his face. "I tracked him down on the Internet – found out that he's still alive. He's down in Rock Ridge … across the street from a grade school."

His personal darkness seems to close in around us. Mr. Kelley stiffens. "All I want to do now … is go down there and kill that bastard!" he spits.

I suddenly feel lost, not expecting and certainly not prepared for this. "Is that something you are planning to do, Mr. Kelley?" I ask, guessing that having a plan or purchasing a weapon might increase the likelihood of violence. Mr. Kelley shifts his gaze out the window again and does not answer. In a moment of near panic, I believe he might actually carry out his threat.

"You know it's not a good idea," I blurt out, not knowing if confrontation is the right thing to do. "In the long run, it won't make you any happier."

He sits silently for a long moment, his eyes focused somewhere far away. My pulse pounds in my ears as I watch his face intently. Finally, he takes a deep breath, looks down at the floor, and says, "No, I suppose not."

I relax a little, but I am not ready to trust that the situation has been diffused so quickly. "Is it all right with you if I call your anger management therapist and tell her about this?" I ask, extremely thankful that I have solid backup already in place.

Mr. Kelley squirms where he sits on the examination table, as if the thought of anyone else knowing makes him very uncomfortable. Finally, the internal struggle ends. "Sure, I guess. I guess that's okay."

"Good. Let me do that right now."

I step out of the room and a wave of fatigue causes me to sag against the wall. Intense emotions vie for recognition. I feel anger at the abuser, sorrow for Mr. Kelley, apprehension about his dangerous rage, and disbelief that we have been running circles around the central issue of this man's life for as long as I have known him.

I take a few slow, deep breaths and try to regain my composure. Was there any way of avoiding this crisis by getting to the truth sooner? Mr. Kelley's defenses had obviously been strong, but sadly, I realize I never asked any probing questions that might have helped him tell his story.

I push up from the wall, vowing to take more diligent and courageous social and sexual histories from now on. While I may not get a full account right away, I owe it to Mr. Kelley and every other hidden abuse survivor to at least start the conversation.

I need to make a phone call. With the right diagnosis, we can finally start the process of healing.

17

The Face of Cancer

John G. Scott, MD, PhD, and Patrick Crommett

The Doctor's Story

Giving patients bad news is never easy, but with Christmas two days away, I had to tell a patient and friend that his seizures were caused by lung cancer metastatic to his brain. I thought about Patrick's remarkable life as I walked down the hospital corridor to his room.

At age 13, Patrick received a dance scholarship with the Joffrey Ballet Company. He finished high school at 16 and moved to New York City as a Joffrey apprentice. Patrick became a solo dancer with the Royal Winnipeg Ballet, and later with the Royal Swedish Ballet in Stockholm. Eventually, tired of the rigors of the professional dancer's life, he moved back to rural Arkansas where he had lived as an infant. He taught ballet to children and helped Steve, his partner of 22 years, create and run the Northeast Arkansas Regional AIDS Network.

Entering the hospital room, I saw Patrick sitting up in bed, with Steve in a chair close by. From the devastated expression on their faces, I immediately knew that the oncologist had already delivered my news. He had informed Patrick that he had three months to live and told them to enjoy this Christmas because it would be their last together. Appalled by his insensitivity, but privately agreeing, I tried to repair the damage. "Take one day at a time. No one can predict when you are going to die. There is always room for hope." I could not let them go home for Christmas without some words of comfort.

In my office a few days later Patrick said, "If I have 1% of a 1% chance of beating this, I want to try." Steve, Patrick's partner, was not doing well. HIV infection, severe hypertension, heart disease and several minor strokes kept him in and out of the hospital. Patrick was determined to stay alive to care for Steve. I had concerns about the wisdom of aggressive therapy, but I arranged for Patrick to see an oncologist who would help him arrive at a treatment plan. I did not anticipate how aggressive that plan would be.

Patrick underwent a needle lung biopsy, which collapsed his lung and gave him a chest tube, but did not produce a tissue diagnosis. Brain surgery followed – again, no tissue diagnosis. A second needle lung biopsy finally made the diagnosis: squamous cell carcinoma. Another brain surgery left him with a mild expressive dysphasia and loss of fine motor control of his left (dominant) hand. Next came chest surgery with removal of the right upper lobe of his lung. A follow-up brain CT scan showed two new brain tumors, requiring whole-brain radiation therapy. A CT scan of the chest showed tumor in the lymph nodes. Chemotherapy failed to slow the tumor growth. Radiation therapy to the chest was the last resort.

Throughout this horrific course of treatment Patrick remained convinced that he would be cured. I was initially convinced that he was undergoing this terrible suffering for nothing. Gradually, though, Patrick's optimism infected me. I began to believe, contrary to everything I knew about his medical prognosis, that Patrick was healing. In my conversations with his other treating physicians, I got the distinct impression that we all felt we were witnessing a medical miracle. Indeed we were. Patrick is alive and well, four years from his diagnosis, with no evidence of cancer.

The Patient's Story

On Thanksgiving Day, Steve and I went to his brother's house for dinner. Sitting on the couch after dinner, my lip started to tremble. My face drew up and my arm shook. It was over within a minute. Everyone thought I was having a stroke, and that made sense to me, because I have not taken the best care of myself. A CT scan showed a little black spot that the emergency room doctor thought was a broken blood vessel. Three weeks later I had a longer seizure, and this time the CT scan showed the spot had tripled in size. I had a bunch of tests, and then a doctor I didn't know walked in and announced that I had cancer of the brain and that it had metastasized. I didn't know what the heck he was talking about. I wasn't familiar with anything pertaining to cancer. He proceeded to tell me that I had approximately two to three months to live and then turned around to leave the room. He stopped at the door, turned back and said, "I hope you two have a good Christmas; it will be your last." This knocked the whey out of me! Steve and I were in a state of shock.

I have traveled a long road from that terrible evening, and I want to share some of the things I learned about myself and about the people who cared for me.

John, as my family doctor, was a sustaining presence. His compassion meant everything to me. He seemed to know what to say to direct me, to help me see what I might do. He never once said, "Patrick, I think you are going to live," but by the same token he was willing to let me be positive about it. That was invaluable. But all medical professionals really count. One of the neatest people I remember was the nurse in the ICU after my lung surgery. She was so positive and vibrant that I couldn't allow myself to be negative around her, and that was really vital to me. I wish that every physician, for just a day, could be in the same kind of situation and be dealt with as Mr Jones or Mrs Smith and experience how patients like me are trying so desperately to hang on to just a tad of hope.

My spirituality and faith were so much a part of my healing. Every artist I have known has a deep, intrinsic spirituality. It may not be a religious attitude, but still a belief in an energy, a strength, a God that is omnipotent. I arrived at a point where I had to say, "Dear Lord, I beg you. I don't have control of my life. Please, please help me through this." From that point on, I felt that the cancer was not going to do me in. There were things I was still supposed to accomplish.

One evening during my chemotherapy I was sitting in my living room feeling like a lump. I remembered having some of my mother's paints out in the garage. I can't explain why I wanted them; I had never painted before. Steve brought in the supplies, and I started painting. After the first day, I felt there was something emerging from the canvas that was not part of me. It was a face, a disturbing face; so disturbing in fact, that I asked Steve to take it away. I didn't want it in the house. A year later, I decided to try painting again. I went to the shed to look for a brush, and there was that face staring at me. I spoke to it, and said, "I'm going to take you in the house, complete you, and then burn you!" I felt so strongly that the face was my cancer. I did finish it, but I didn't burn it (*see* Figure 1).

That painting opened a whole new world for me. I think the radiation or surgery or both were mind altering. I began to see forms, beasts, and faces in trees and flowers. I began painting what I saw. Painting has become a great joy and a cleansing, purging tool for me. Someone commented about one of my landscapes, "I love that because I feel like I can walk into it." And I said, "I can." I can stare and see visions in clouds and trees and dawns and dusks. The colors are luminescent. Everything is brighter than it used to be. I have a whole new way of looking at everything. I look at something and see the importance of it to all of us, be it a

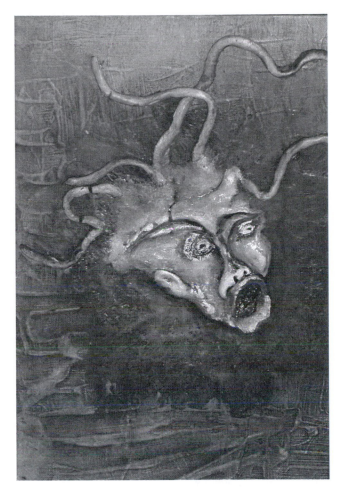

FIGURE 1 "The Face of Cancer," by Patrick Crommett

bush or a plant or a person. I was so unaware of what a wonderful gift each day is. It can be pouring down rain, and I'm overwhelmed with joy to be alive on such a gorgeous day. These have been powerful gifts of this cancer.

The cancer has been a gift in other ways, as well. My spirituality deepened, and my relationship with my daughter strengthened tremendously. When Steve became extremely ill, I prayed that we could get him through one more time, but the cancer helped me recognize that the time had come to let go of him. He was suffering and in pain, and one night I sat on the bed, held him by the hand and said, "Steve, I know you're holding on with everything you have for me. Don't worry about me. I will be OK. If you need to, just let go." He said, "Thank you, Patrick." Two days later, he died. I think all of us have a tendency to be selfish about losing those we love. We forget that one of the greatest gifts of our lives is to be able to let go.

The cancer left me with a tremor of my left hand. I can no longer write with my left hand, nor play the piano. I have always been a terrific turner in dance. I can't turn worth a flip anymore. I have no balance. I miss the abilities that cancer has taken from me, but it has given more than taken. In retrospect, I view it as a wake-up call. I know I have been blessed, and come what may, if I dropped dead tomorrow, I have had miraculous happenings in my life, and a wonderful, wonderful life.

Epilogue

From the worldview of the biomedical model of disease, Patrick should be dead. To quote Patrick, "The doctors were stunned at the amount of time I had survived. In fact, a physician said, 'Patrick, we are flying by the seat of our pants. We don't understand at all why you are reacting so positively to everything we are doing.'"

Patrick and I learned the limitations of that biomedical model. He could not have survived without the sophisticated medical treatment he received, but that treatment was insufficient to explain the healing that took place in his body and spirit. And in mine. Healing works in both directions. Patrick taught me to trust my intuition as well as my medical knowledge. In my relationship with him, I experienced the healing power of hope and learned to think about possibility rather than prognosis. During home visits to Patrick and Steve in the final days of Steve's life, I was powerfully affected by their love and commitment. That witness helped me reevaluate my own priorities in relationship to my family and my work.

This is more than a story about illness. It is a story about transcendence of illness, and the value of instinct and faith and trust in the relationship between a doctor and patient, and how these combined in a mysterious way to produce the healing process we found in each other.

Section 4

Connections

In our suffering and our joy we are connected to one another with unbreakable and compelling human bonds.

—Rachel Naomi Remen, MD[1]

Our connections – the links that join person to person and heart to heart – enrich our lives. It is through a sense of connection that we find meaning, experience love, and share our pleasures and pains. Family medicine is a unique incubator for human connection because it is medicine that spans a lifetime. Together, patients and physicians deal with intimate aspects of human existence: the routine yet wondrous evolution from child to adult to elder, and the extraordinary experiences of birth, illness, death, and disease.

This section explores some of the enduring elements on which human connection is built.

- *Humanity*: what is the physician's role in helping patients change themselves and their lives? For family physician David Loxterkamp, the answer is found in the humanity we share and the relationships that connect us.
- *Friendship*: when Renate Justin met her newborn patient Ruth she had no idea they would develop a decades-long relationship that would shape her life and medical practice.
- *Compassion*: meaningful relationships are not always long-lived. Sara Shields reflects on a brief, heartbreaking encounter with a patient and the bittersweet bond that connects them.

- *Communication*: a physician's ability to improvise when talking with a patient helps their partnership flourish. For physician and jazz aficionado Paul Haidet, jazz improvisation offers important lessons for patient-physician communication.
- *Inspiration*: Steve Blevins has always enjoyed seeing Jerry, his longtime patient. However, when Steve experiences a major life change, Jerry becomes a touch-stone and an inspiration.

Reference

1. Remen RN. *Kitchen Table Wisdom*. New York, NY: Riverhead Books; 1996. p. 140.

18

A Change Will Do You Good

David Loxterkamp, MD

*It is not the strongest of the species that survives, nor the most intel-
ligent, but the one most responsive to change.*

—Clarence Darrow[1]

Notes While Waiting

Change comes slowly to a small town. The tides rise and fall, seasons turn, the
newborn nursery and the grounds of Mt. Repose Cemetery form bookends in
a natural balance. Nary a brick has been added or subtracted to our downtown
since the Great Conflagration of 1869. Pleasant chatter at the Beano Hall,
Thompson's Barbershop, or deli counter at Hannaford's drifts ineluctably toward
sports, kids, and illness. And the census has not budged for a century and a half,
though employment shifted from shipbuilding to shoe manufacturing to poultry
processing to telemarketing, tourism, and the service sector.

I am part of that sector. For 23 years I have cared for an endless stream of
knotted joints, nagging coughs, and niggling doubts of a rural patient panel that
has aged imperceptibly in the watch of their aging physician. Then one day, a
death or diagnosis changes everything. In its wake, the patient and family doctor
struggle to patch their shattered world. When I began the practice of medicine,
I was drawn to the high-decibel drama of life: birth and death, emergencies, and
intensive care. But I have come to appreciate the more delicate and nuanced
branch points: where the most dramatic change is our realization the world

around us has moved on. We must choose between living in the present or locking ourselves in the past.

Change of Life

Patients often enter crossroads where obvious decisions abound: quit smoking or it will kill you; leave the abusive relationship or crazy job before it is too late; risk a total hip replacement while you can still survive and enjoy it. These are questions I dance around each day. But a sharper thorn digs my side: why do some patients grasp for help while others are swept past, beyond reach, isolated in their self-destruction and despair?

The agencies of timing and luck confound my search for more consistent clues. I do not so much orchestrate change as listen closely for it. William Miller and Stephen Rollnick see the process of change through a framework they call motivational interviewing. Their work is indebted to the client-centered approach of Carl Rogers. It is less technique than a manner of communication that seeks to spring clients from the trap of indecision. For the patient facing a choice, as doctors see it, other options compete. Only the patient can resolve his ambivalence by choosing among them. And resolution takes time. Empathic clinicians can offer their time, space, self-awareness, and self-confidence, and they recognize that the patient's resistance to change is often a reflection of the doctor's own haste and indelicacy. When commitment to change finally comes, Miller and Rollnick assert, it is always a positive choice:

> People don't change because they haven't suffered enough. Constructive behavior change seems to arise when the person connects it with something of intrinsic value, something important, something cherished. People often get stuck, not because they fail to appreciate the downside of their situation, but because they feel at least two ways about it. The way out of the forest has to do with exploring and following what the person is experiencing and what, from his or her perspective, truly matters.[2]

The Patient

I am called to the Emergency Department to admit Mr V, a 52-year-old truck driver with unstable angina. The physician on duty carefully noted the progressive symptoms of chest tightness, shortness of breath, and sweating during the previous week. Intravenous metoprolol, subcutaneous enoxaparin, and four chewable baby aspirin were given in timely fashion. New-onset diabetes was documented, along with the strong recommendation that the patient be hospitalized for observation, provocative cardiac testing, and diabetes education and treatment.

What the doctor failed to record was a pending court date, scheduled for the following Tuesday, to resolve a neighbor's complaint against the noise and pollution of the patient's rock quarry. Nor did he document a notice by the Department of Environmental Protection that they intended to investigate the complaint. Or the 12- to 16-hour days the patient had been working to make ends meet. Or the anxiety attacks and insomnia that resulted, and the Michelob Lite he drank to calm his nerves. How does a beaten brow or oil-stained work cloths skew our judgment of a patient's capacity for change?

In the corner, a woman – his wife – wipes tears from her eyes as I talk about the blessing that these events can sometimes bring, the chance to look at our lives and reorder priorities. She takes me aside and whispers that a similar episode occurred last year; his left arm went numb and weak for several days but improved before she could convince him to see the doctor.

What will happen after the acute coronary syndrome has been ruled out and his blood glucose returns to normal? This question in its varied expressions has absorbed me for more than two decades. The scientific method is no match for the barrage and blare of problems I face in the social arena. Patients live and work within social groups that explain their illness and provide the motivation to rise above it. Doctors, inside our own social enclave, develop treatment goals that drift away from the patients' base of reference. Thus it is possible for a manufacturer to claim therapeutic advantage for a drug that improves biomarkers and disease-specific mortality but worsens the quality of life and overall death rate.

In the 1950s, the Hungarian-born psychoanalyst Michael Balint coined the term patient-centered care, thus turning the focus of professional concern and scrutiny back on the patient's social context. Balint's other great contribution was to imaginatively explore the role of the doctor as drug. He saw that clinicians could just as easily contribute positively or negatively to a reciprocal therapeutic relationship. Work with groups of general practitioners at the Tavistock Clinic (London) culminated in his seminal work, *The Doctor, His Patient, and the Illness*, in 1958.[3] This book had a profound effect on the training of primary care physicians, even in the United States, where it has been said:

> No factor has influenced the evolving nature of family medicine more profoundly than its ties to the behavioral sciences. And no work has

exemplified this link more trenchantly than Balint's *The Doctor, His Patient, and the Illness.*[4]

Balint groups are established in nearly one-half of the family medicine residency programs in the United States. An overreaching goal is to challenge each physician with the question, "What kind of doctor do I need to be for this patient today?" In addition to promoting awareness in the doctor-patient relationship, there is also an element of self-help. Jonathan Gore, a Balint group leader, sees these groups as a way of helping physicians treat difficult patients without resorting to those human defenses that tend to distance or denigrate. The hope is that young doctors could cope with caring for difficult patients while maintaining their own equanimity and mental health.

Like my seasoned colleagues, I know that the doctor-patient relationship is both a gold mine and a land mine, a source of gratitude and pride, a bounty of inside secrets about the requirements for human survival and the costs of caring for those who suffer. Change is not a solo flight. People in crisis need companionship and guidance. They often need another to shift their gaze from the conflict at hand to its unconscious origins. They need assurance that the shift is not only possible but worth the effort.

A Life of Change

I recently returned to part-time teaching after 15 years in private practice. It has been edifying and humbling to supervise residents who have so readily mastered the medical corpus. What could I teach them about the care of patients in a setting (the family medicine center) that self-selects for some of the most difficult and marginalized I have ever encountered? How could I convey what my patients have taught me, or what I learned by living in one place for two decades, or what marriage and children and life and death have hewn in my bones? What could be said in a 5-minute consultation that does not ring of cheap anecdote and sentimentality? I found myself repeating a few whispered warnings that spared me from many an unseen but ever-present danger.

First, command the science that underpins our authority. Yet, understand that – in the words of Kafka – "to write prescriptions is easy, but to come to an understanding of people is hard."[5]

Second, understand that patients who insist "you're the doctor" are here for themselves. Offer them a mirror, or better, a portrait painted in layers by an unhurried listener who works in oils of word and touch. But the artist must know his footing, as Anais Nin warns: "We don't see things as they are, we see things as we are."[6]

Third, realize that good advice is as worthless as all the prescriptions written to quell our insecurity or deflect the patient's inscrutable complaints. Most patients change when life-altering diagnoses compel them to or when years of self-neglect begin to take their toll. It is then that we can probe again for the shifts in awareness or readiness for change.

Change in others is beside our control. So we do what we can: order tests, prescribe drugs, and perform procedures – necessary or not – that prove our good intentions. We offer a hand of friendship. Patient care is more than a series of transactions, an accountant's log of money exchanged for itemized service. At every step it harbors the chance to express tolerance, affection, weakness, and commonality. Broken, confused patients seek a stronger ally; the doctor, in turn, recognizes himself in their illness.

It is through the open door of relationship that a new kind of authority emerges, at once personal and deeply moral, one that offers honesty as an invitation instead of a demand. I have practiced long enough to know that my actions have lasting consequences, intended or not, with or without legal or ethical aftershocks. I am forever bound to my patients, my wounds alloyed to theirs. There was never a more sensitive and astute observer of this stage in a doctor's career than the poet-laureate William Carlos Williams. He was keenly aware of the flawed human being he threw at his patients, prompting Robert Coles to remark of him that "presumptuousness and self-importance are the wounds this life imposes upon those privy to the wounds of others," and later, remarking himself, "There's nothing like a difficult patient to show us ourselves."[7]

Return

Mr V reappeared one late afternoon, six weeks after his hospital discharge. Little surprise that his stress echocardiogram was normal and his morning blood glucose readings, jotted on a legal pad, clustered around 100 mg/dL. Mr V was relieved to report that the lawsuit was dismissed. He returned to driving a truck with its attendant 14-hour days. I met the eyes of his wife, as they once met in the Emergency Department. We both felt the window of opportunity shimmy down. Though a change might have done him good, Mr V is alive, and so am I. We are working still, and putting our trust in the strength of a handshake.

I don't know what change I had hoped for, or on what criteria I might have judged it. Perhaps we will meet again at another crossroads. Change takes time, and is meted out in the mutuality of human relationship – where the doctor and patient cling to a common log on the rising river.

References

1. Darrow, C. *The Quality of Life for the Black Elderly: Challenges and Opportunities: Hearing before the Select Committee on Aging, House of Representatives, One Hundredth Congress, first session.* September 25, 1987. http://en.wikiquote.org/wiki/Clarence_Darrow.
2. Miller W, Rollnick S. *Motivational Interviewing: Preparing People for Change.* New York, NY: Guilford Press; 2002. p. 12.
3. Balint M. *The Doctor, His Patient and the Illness.* London: Pitman Publishing Co; 1957.
4. Johnson AH. The Balint movement in America. *Fam Med.* 2001; 33(3): 174–77.
5. Kafka F. A country doctor. In: *Selected Short Stories of Franz Kafka.* New York, NY: The Modern Library; 1952. p. 252.
6. Attributed to Anais Nin. http://en.wikiquote.org/wiki/Anais_Nin.
7. Williams WC, Coles R (compiler). *The Doctor Stories.* New York, NY: New Directions; 1984. p. xiii.

19

Linking Ruth to Her Past

Renate G. Justin, MD

TOWARD THE END OF MY CAREER AS A FAMILY PHYSICIAN, I WORKED for a health maintenance organization. In this medical care system, I could not be with my patients during times of crisis. If they were acutely ill and hospitalized, a hospitalist attended them. We did not share in the joys of life, birth, or recovery from a serious illness, nor did we share in tragedies, death, or disability. My relationship with my patients was friendly and respectful, but not intimate.

At the beginning of my practice as a family physician, 50 years ago, my relationship with my patients was quite different. I cared for several generations of the same family. I looked after some patients from birth to death. Some encounters with patients lasted 10 minutes, other were much longer; some were preponderantly objective and scientific, during others our souls touched. This subtle interplay of objective and subjective responses required an ability to listen, to divine what the specific meeting of the doctor and patient demanded. The relationships between my patients and myself varied as the colors on the artist's palate.

My relationship with Ruth evolved over three decades. Ruth and I first met when I attended her birth and then when her grandmother brought her to the office for delayed immunizations. Ruth's mother died in the early 1960s of breast cancer when Ruth was not quite two years old. Ruth's paternal grandmother moved in with her son to look after her little granddaughter. The well-child checkup was uneventful; Ruth was a cuddly baby with the same big brown eyes that had graced her mother's face. I inquired about the grandmother's well-being, and she said, "Ruth is keeping me alive; without her I wouldn't be here."

I saw Ruth for her school physical examination when she was five years old. It was hard to believe the cute baby had reached school age. She was fine, pretty with long dark hair; she looked like her mom. She also was smart, and I predicted accurately that she would do well in school. She no longer suffered acutely from the deprivation caused by her mother's death; she had bonded well to her grandmother. I stopped worrying about who would nurture this little girl and shepherd her through her teenage years. I sent her off with a hug and "enjoy school."

The next visit was for a sports physical. We were becoming better acquainted, and I knew that Ruth trusted me when she asked about birth control, a subject her grandmother found difficult to discuss. My own children were close to Ruth in age, and I felt protective and motherly toward her, especially as her grandmother was aging.

When I filled out college forms about her past and present health history, Ruth and I began to talk about her genetic predisposition to breast cancer. I took care of her mother and three aunts who died of this disease. Ruth thought her maternal grandmother, whom I did not know, also died at a young age of breast cancer. I taught Ruth self-breast examination, and we discussed the need for frequent office visits to allow me to check her breasts. We also weighed the option of bilateral mastectomies, but Ruth rejected this choice, saying, "I want to have children and want to be able nurse them." I wished that I owned a genetic wand that I could wave over her.

Ruth's father remarried and moved to another town. Her biyearly office visits did not raise concern. Ruth graduated from college, and her grandmother died during the same week. We saw each other frequently during the following months and talked about Ruth's great loss. I was now the female adult in her life who had known her longer than any one, and the only one who had known her family. We mourned not only Ruth's grandmother, but also her mother, whom I remembered as possessing quietude and the surety that comes with inner peace. Ruth was much like her. During this time of sadness, we had long talks and frequent telephone calls. I respected Ruth. She managed on her own after her grandmother's death and in due time became joyful and optimistic. When she visited the office, she greeted each of us with a warm smile and "Hi, Freda, how is your Mom?" or "Rita, does your little one walk yet?"

Ruth and her fiancé came in for premarital serologic tests. Tom, whom she met in college, was an accountant. I liked him. We discussed birth control, but Ruth and Tom desired to have children soon. I sent a card on their first wedding anniversary. Not long after, when Ruth called, my receptionist interrupted me. She had detected panic in Ruth's voice. I picked up the telephone and knew what had happened before Ruth told me. I asked her to come to the office without delay. She was crying when I entered the examination room, and I used a tissue to dry her tears and then gave her the box. My palpation confirmed Ruth's findings – there was a mass in her left breast, small, but hard. I felt no nodes but was as apprehensive as Ruth. I had a clear sense of déjà vu. How long ago was it that I had felt a similar mass in Ruth's mother's breast? We talked, picked a surgeon, and got an appointment in the afternoon.

I arrived at the hospital early the morning of surgery and found Tom sitting on Ruth's bed holding her in his embrace. They both had been crying. I fought to keep my own tears from spilling, yet I resisted the impulse to be reassuring when I could not find cause for optimism. I was no longer an objective observer of this tragedy, I had become an engaged participant.

Ruth had a radical mastectomy, and after surgery I spent many hours with her and Tom explaining the most recent protocol for breast cancer and how it would influence fertility, longevity, and quality of life. We also grieved together. After months of intravenous chemotherapy, hospitalizations for staphylococcal infections in her left arm, and radiation, Ruth's menses resumed, and she and Tom were soon anticipating the birth of their first child. They were ecstatic. I felt like a happy grandparent, but worried and anxious. I knew the statistics only too well.

When little Frank arrived, we were relieved that he was a healthy baby boy. Ruth and Tom named him after me and his other grandmothers. I saw them often. Tom always came to the office with Frank and Ruth. Frank was only two years old when we discovered that Ruth's cancer had recurred. Ruth was angry that she had to die young – she was only in her late 20s – that she wasted the months of treatment, nausea, and misery, and as she said, "it did no good."

We now were friends, and I no longer wore a white coat when I visited Ruth at home. Her house was located on a lake, and we sat on its shore together watching the fish jump and the ducks teach their young how to swim. The concern of the ducks for their ducklings caused Ruth to weep. "Who will teach my duckling how to walk, to swim?" She made me promise over and over that I would not abandon Tom and Frank after she died. We embraced as I left, both of us aware that our time together was short. As I drove home, I allowed myself to sob. My friend was dying, and there was no way to delay the inevitable.

During the funeral I held Frank in my arms; he wanted to play in the grass, run around. I reflected on my first friendly, but distant "hello" to Ruth as a tiny infant, and my tearful "good-bye" to my close friend. I saw Tom and Frank regularly until Frank was ready to start school. By that time, Tom had found a partner, and their beautiful new home was at a distance from where Ruth was buried.

Would Ruth's life have been different today, now that geneticists have identified the familial breast cancer gene that can deplete the women in a family? I do not think so. I believe that Ruth would have rejected genetic testing; she wanted to remain hopeful.

Knowing Ruth over decades, in joy and despair, inevitably formed strong ties between us. My relationship with her included being a physician, a substitute parent, a grandparent, and at the end, a friend. I did not hesitate to fill these roles. By allowing my feelings to be expressed, I enriched my own experience as a physician; at the same time, I ministered to Ruth's, my patient's, needs.

As a physician I was taught to keep emotionally distant from my patients so I could maintain the best therapeutic milieu. I "have been trained in medicine to believe that subjectivity is the enemy of science – even truth."[1] Ruth and I could not maintain distance, especially at the end of her life. At that moment friendship, closeness rather than distance, was likely more therapeutic because it recognized our common humanity.

It was the experience of being present in different roles in Ruth's as well as in her family's life for many years that made being her family physician humbling and rewarding.

Reference

1. Cassel EJ. *The Healers Art*. Philadelphia, Penn: JB Lippincott Co; 1976. p. 105.

20

On This Day of Mothers and Sons

Sara G. Shields, MD, MS

THE MORNING BEGINS IN CELEBRATION, MY SON BRIGHTLY LEAPING awake in joyful anticipation of his eighth birthday unfolding before him. This day will truly be his. Before work, I share the merriment of his breakfast birthday gifts and then kiss him good-bye more wistfully than usual. My happiness at his excitement is tinged both with memory of his newborn self so fleetingly long ago and with sadness at departing for work. This day should be fully his – and fully mine to be there as I was at the beginning. But he seems unaware and is too busy thinking about his latest Lego and his upcoming party to give me more than a quick airborne hug.

At work, I, too, become busy thinking about other things, enveloped in the tumult of my overbooked schedule at a community health center. After a couple of patients do not show, I have a breather to finish notes in a chart at the nurses' station. When our obstetric nurse-practitioner approaches me, I expect her usual quick curbside question about a newly pregnant woman's medication list or yesterday's telephone messages. But she is somber and succinct as she hands me her Doptone. "I'm seeing a woman at 30 weeks' with no fetal movement for a week and no fetal heart tones now." I put down my pen immediately to follow her. Somehow in her tone and my response, we both wordlessly know that if she cannot find the heartbeat, I probably cannot either.

I enter the examination room and introduce myself to the woman sitting on the examination table. She's Salvadoran, quiet with respect for doctors, neatly dressed, and carefully coiffed. Her prenatal history is unremarkable; her

2-year-old daughter is at home while her sister-in-law dropped her off for this visit. She knows this baby is a boy – she paid for a sonogram to know that.

I ask a few questions about her history and symptoms as I wash my hands; I query again about when she last felt movement and explain that I will also try to listen for the baby. In these first few moments of meeting each other, I cannot quite read her face. I wonder silently what kept her from calling sooner than this regularly scheduled appointment and what she thinks could be wrong.

I put my hands gently on her soft belly, feeling for her uterus and the baby's position before I reach for the Doptone. Under my hands, her fundus is soft, the baby still. I listen in the usual places, moving the Doptone around, searching for the swift swishing sound of life's pulse, but hearing only static. The nurse-practitioner knocks on the door to tell me that luckily for us our sonography technician is available immediately. I look this mother in the eye and make a swift decision to be completely honest right now: I say in my pretty good but not perfect Spanish, "Well, sometimes we can't hear the heartbeat because of the way the baby is lying, with his back to your back, so we need to get an ultrasound to check for sure; and sometimes, when you haven't felt him and we can't hear him, that may mean the baby's died."

Her face, expectant on mine, crumples as she gasps at these words. I so swiftly, desperately want to take them back. Why have I said this now, before the sonogram? Maybe I'm wrong? Why am I taking away any hope now with these blunt, harsh words? Maybe I should have used an interpreter? And yet part of me knows that somehow in her almost unreadable gaze she already knows, even as she still hopes.

In the sonography room, the technician moves the transducer around, searching, and we wait, looking at the machine, hoping. Our silence merely voices the certainty of what we are about to say. If there were a heartbeat, wouldn't we be instantly telling her, showing her, reassuring her with our relieved smiles? In our hesitation, she knows the final truth, reads it in our quiet unsmiling faces. She gasps and sobs anew as I turn to her and repeat now, with this photographic certainty, what I already said – "Your baby has died. I am so, so sorry." My voice trails off. I touch her hand and let her cry, her sobs shaking the grainy ultrasound view as the technician tries to finish her pictures. I don't think the technician wanted her to know quite yet, but I can't let her wait longer. "I am so sorry," I say again.

The long walk back to the examination room is eerie. I suggest a moment to collect ourselves as the walk takes us through two crowded waiting rooms. I know the spectacle we make – not the expected joy of pregnancy but rather a red-eyed pregnant woman with somber companions. Back in the examination room, with a box of tissues at hand, she meets my gaze with simple questions, the ones I'm waiting for – "Why? What now?" She wants to call her husband, her sister-in-law. I hold her hand, I tell her in broad terms some of her options. I tell her for now there are no answers, but some will come. I tell her this is not her fault. I tell her again how sorry I am. I spend most of the rest of my morning with her.

I teach residents how to do this telling, I've read about how to do it, I've watched videos, I've had advice from other faculty and heard their wisdom, I've even had to deliver such news a few other times in my career. Yet right now, in the agony of this woman's experience, on this day that began for me with celebrating my own mothering moments, I feel so very deeply the blunt, hard pain of this mother, this moment of knowing death. I am the one who has to move those shocking diagnostic words out of their sticking place in my throat to tell her news that I, as a mother, know is unfathomably agonizing. When I tell such news in the future, it will never be with the distance of protocols or practiced professional phrases, but always with my personal awareness of the boundless depth of maternal love and the inextricable potential for maternal suffering. Indeed, this day teaches me again how interwoven are my personal knowledge of human connections and my professional work with families.

Later this day I talk with this woman's primary care physician, a resident, herself on duty that evening. I tell her I'm on my way to my son's birthday party, and she exclaims, "Today is my son's birthday too!" So here we are: the grieving woman, her primary doctor, and the doctor this woman didn't know before today. We are all mothers who have felt baby sons kick within us. Today, two of us celebrate our sons' growth and life, always remembering those movements. The third one of us, whose unborn son no longer kicks within, will grieve always, remembering this day.

21

Jazz and the "Art" of Medicine

Improvisation in the Medical Encounter

Paul Haidet, MD, MPH

Intro

> *The thing that sets Roy apart from other musicians is that he listens so well. He teaches you to listen carefully and to respond accordingly, to put things in perspective, not to simply go out for yourself.*
>
> —Pianist McCoy Tyner, describing drummer Roy Haynes[1]

Communication is central to human experience. It provides the vehicle through which we share ideas, coordinate actions, and build social structures.[2] In medicine, important care processes such as information sharing and decision making occur in the context of patient-physician communication.[3] A large and growing body of research shows that high-quality communication results in fewer medical errors, lower rates of litigation, and a variety of favorable social, psychological, and biological outcomes.[4–12]

Improvisation is an important aspect of patient-physician communication. The medical encounter, like most encounters involving communication, is typically unscripted and constructed "in the moment."[13] Although physicians often follow biomedical patterns of inquiry,[14] a patient-centered care ideal calls for adjustments to and departures from these patterns in response to concerns and perspectives voiced by the patient.[15] In other words, physicians often need to improvise when they encounter patients' unique illness narratives.[16] Improvisation guides a physician's process of making moment-to-moment communicative decisions (e.g., what to say next, how to structure particular questions, which threads to follow, when to interrupt and when to let the patient keep going). Stephen Nachmanovitch, PhD, a violinist and scholar on creativity and the spiritual underpinnings of art, described a tension between biomedical training and patients' novel contexts as he discussed the importance of improvisation in medicine:

> In *real* medicine you view the person as unique – in a sense you drop your training. You are immersed in the case itself, letting your view of it develop in context. You certainly use your training; you refer to it, understand it, ground yourself in it, but you don't allow your training to blind you to the actual person who is sitting in front of you. In this way, you pass beyond competence to *presence*. To do anything artistically, you have to acquire technique, but you create *through* your technique and not *with* it.[17]

As a communication educator and researcher, former disc jockey, and amateur jazz historian, I often marvel at the many parallels between jazz and medicine. For example, understanding jazz history can also enhance one's understanding of many modern medical issues. These issues include racial disparities, as experienced by cornetists Louis Armstrong and Bix Beiderbecke; the life-world of addiction, as embodied by saxophonist Charlie Parker; and leadership skills, as practiced by bandleaders such as Duke Ellington, Art Blakey, and others. Several scholars have used jazz to describe insights about organizational development[18,19] and the practice of evidence-based medicine.[13]

Although many characteristics of jazz have analogies in medicine, jazz's central focus on improvisation is particularly relevant to patient-physician communication. Improvisation is the primary vehicle that jazz players use to relate and communicate musically with one another.[20] When describing the improvisational process, many jazz musicians and critics use verbal communication metaphors.[21] For example, jazz musicians will commonly describe a particular performance using phrases such as, "I said this, and then he said that, etc." In this essay, I turn the metaphor around and use jazz improvisation as a lens to explore patient-physician communication. Although such an exploration could take many directions, I focus on communication at 3 levels: (1) as an act, (2) as a trait, and

(3) as an event. For each level, I begin with a description of jazz improvisation and follow with an exploration of the meaning that the description holds for patient-physician communication. Along the way, I suggest particular jazz performances to augment the essay. Listening to the performances, although not critical, will enhance the reading experience by providing an additional illustration of the concepts discussed.

A Communicative Act: Creating Space

> *Man, you don't have to play a whole lot of notes. You just have to play the pretty ones.*
>
> —Trumpeter Miles Davis[22]

During the medical encounter, physicians engage in a number of communicative acts, including question asking, information giving, and supportive talk.[23] Researchers and educators have devised elaborate coding schemes to characterize the content and process of such acts.[24–27] In my experience as a practitioner and teacher, I have found the act of providing communicative space to the patient to be one of the most powerful yet underused skills by physicians.[28]

What is space and how does it relate to jazz or patient-physician communication? When I am in the room with a patient, I sometimes think about how Miles Davis improvised. Miles came of age during the bebop era of jazz, when dominant trumpet players such as Dizzy Gillespie and Fats Navarro played blistering solos in the upper register at breakneck speed. It was said that Miles lacked the technical skill to play like Dizzy or Fats; however, whatever technical ability Miles did or did not have, his brilliance as an improviser manifested itself not so much in what he played as in what he did *not* play. To hear a solo by Miles is to hear space. Miles does not play a lot of notes, he just plays the *right* ones. He conserves notes, plays them at a relaxed pace, plays on the "back end" of the beat, and drops musical hints that allow the listener to use their imagination to fill in the phrases. The effect in songs such as "All Blues" (Columbia/Legacy CD *Kind of Blue*, CK64935) is that it becomes easy to hear not only the solo, but also what the rest of the band is playing. The solo voice gently leads one to hear the sum total of the music – not just the soloist's musical statements way out in front, but those statements within the broader context of the whole band.[29]

As a physician, I strive to use communicative space as Miles did. Rather than take up all the space in the conversation with strings of "yes/no" questions or long physiological explanations, I find that I am at my best when I can give patients space to say what they want to say, using my communications to gently lead patients through a telling of the illness narrative from their perspective, rather than forcing the narrative to follow my biomedical perspective.[30] In this space, patients often either tell their story, allowing me to understand the context around their symptoms, or ask the questions that allow me to tailor my explanations to their unique concerns. Unfortunately, in our culture, we are not generally comfortable with pauses or quiet. When the situation is compounded by the chaos of a busy clinic, it becomes difficult to remain focused and open to the directions that patients take us. For most practitioners, space does not come naturally; it takes practice and discipline to develop.[31]

Because space is multidimensional, it is a complex concept to research or teach. It requires attention to both communicative and narrative parameters. Communicative parameters include not only silence (as measured by metrics such as total physician and patient talk time), but also latency (the time between the end of the patient's statements and the beginning of the physician's statements) and pace (the number of words one utters per minute). Narrative parameters include care in the application of redirections (e.g., interruptions, changes in the subject) and specific attention to communicative constraints placed on the patient (e.g., the yes/no constraint inherent in closed-ended questions). When practitioners effectively use space, paying attention to both communicative and narrative parameters in the conversation, patients do not feel pressured or forced to omit information from their story.[32] Rather, they are freed up to describe their health concerns on their own terms.[33–35]

A Communicative Trait: Developing Voice

After the jazzman has learned the fundamentals of his instrument and the traditional techniques of jazz ... he must then "find himself," must be reborn, must find, as it were, his soul. He must achieve, in short, his self-determined identity.

—Ralph Ellison[36]

An important task for young jazz improvisers is to develop their voice. Learning musical theory, gaining familiarity with jazz scales and chord structures, mastering an instrument, apprenticing in the real world, and learning the repertoire of common songs are all important milestones; however, these alone are not enough to achieve musical success. Although the knowledge and skills are essential, the jazz musicians who eventually achieve critical and historical impact are those who channel the theory, technique, and ideas of their predecessors through their own personalities, feelings, and experiences. In this way, they develop a sound that is fresh and original in a process often called *developing one's voice*. This process requires curiosity, self-reflection, a clear and frequently revisited sense of purpose, and attention to the musical contexts that young musicians find themselves in.[37,38]

An excellent example of the development of improvisational voice is the evolution of saxophonist John Coltrane's playing in the 1950s and 1960s. Through his interactions with mentors such as trumpeter Miles Davis, pianist Thelonious Monk, and others, Coltrane's improvisations went from unexciting interpretations of his era's predominant musical forms to explosive flurries of patterns at speeds so great that the notes seemed to blur together, an effect that fellow musicians and critics came to call *sheets of sound*. Those sheets of sound were a hallmark of Coltrane's unique voice and can be heard on a number of recordings including "Giant Steps," which was recorded in 1959 (Atlantic Records CD *Giant Steps*, 1311-12). Although earlier recordings reveal that Coltrane possessed the technical skill to play sheets of sound as early as 1956, his fully mature voice, with its unique phrasings and idiosyncrasies, did not become evident until years later. During that time, Coltrane was undergoing an intense exploration of his life, his goals, his music, and his spirituality. This exploration translated musically into the development of his unique voice.[39]

Like jazz musicians, physicians need to develop their improvisational voice. Basic communication skills, such as agenda setting, effective use of open- and closed-ended questions, and patient-centered interviewing techniques, remain the building blocks of good communication[40]; these skills are like the scales that a musician must master. Similarly, the common communicative scenarios, such as breaking bad news, counseling for behavior change, and conversing about end-of-life issues, are like the songs that a musician must learn.[41] Learning does not end at the basic skills or patterns of communication, however. Physicians must begin to incorporate knowledge and skills into their own personal style. They must creatively apply this style in each encounter in a way that fits well with the particular context and the communications of the patient. As an example, consider the bad news scenario. Experienced patient-centered doctors do not all break bad news in the same manner,[42] nor do they all rigidly follow generally accepted guidelines[43,44] for breaking bad news. Although there might be points of commonality, patient-centered physicians will do and say things in a manner that honors not only the humanity of the patient, but their own humanity as well. In a sense, these physicians "show up" in the medical encounter, rather than adopting a third-party stance that can act as a barrier to relationship building. Educators and researchers are beginning to realize that a communicative process that honors both patient and physician will strengthen the relationship that develops.[45] Skill, technique, and theory provide a foundation, or point of departure, for a physician to develop his or her voice and bring it to the medical encounter.

A Communicative Event: Cultivating Ensemble

> *Group improvisation is a further challenge. Aside from the weighty technical problem of collective coherent thinking, there is the very human, even social need for sympathy from all members to bend for the common result.*

> —Pianist Bill Evans[46]

Voice is only the beginning, because it takes more than one voice to have a conversation. On the one hand, there is the voice of the soloist. On the other hand, there are the voices of the other band members, who, in great jazz performances, are improvising also. The tension for all players is how much space to take in the music and what to play in that space to support each other's musical statements. If the soloist and other players are not listening to each other, the music sounds disjointed and dissonant, as if they are playing past each other. The early 1960s trio of bandleader-pianist Bill Evans, bassist Scott LaFaro, and drummer Paul Motian showed the jazz world how members of an ensemble could all simultaneously solo and support each other. Evans and LaFaro in particular had developed such a level of mutual respect and empathic listening that there are points during recordings such as "Waltz for Debby" (Riverside CD *Waltz for Debby*, OJCCD-210-2) when it is difficult to discern whose is the solo voice and whose is the supporting one. LaFaro's bass and Evans' piano epitomized the concept of ensemble by building coherent and harmonious improvisational performances out of two individual instruments' statements.[47]

Communication Accommodation Theory (CAT) provides a verbal analogy for ensemble. In CAT, one's statements are viewed in the context of their partner's statements. This contextual view allows one's statements to be classified as either converging to or diverging from the partner's statements. For example, in response to a question, providing an answer that is topically appropriate would be seen as an act of convergence. On the other hand, asking an unrelated question in response to a question (e.g., a doctor asking, "Are you short of breath?" in response to a patient's question, "Is my chest pain serious, doctor?") is an act of divergence.[48] Acts of convergence and divergence influence the patient-physician relationship, because converging statements signify a desire to gain approval, affiliate, establish rapport, and communicate meaning effectively, whereas diverging statements aim to separate, exert control, and generally downplay the statements of the partner.

Physicians and patients can achieve ensemble in their improvisation by accommodating, where possible, to each others' statements and styles of communication. Although our prevailing culture generally positions the physician as the leader of the conversation, ideally, the medical encounter would be characterized by voices that exist in harmony, rather than one striving to dominate the other.[49,50] A collective ensemble improvisation is therefore characterized by the physician's, patient's, and sometimes other voices making assertions, listening to what others have to say, supporting each other, and incorporating each others' ideas into a common understanding.[30,34] This back-and-forth communication is critical for the physician's understanding of the patient's illness perspective and for the patient's understanding of the biomedical processes underlying the illness and the therapies that medicine has to offer.[51] Ensemble improvisation is the process that makes shared decision making possible, because it allows all voices to find common ground about the decisions to be made.[52]

What does it take for physicians to enter into ensemble with patients? As implied by the previous quotes from McCoy Tyner and Bill Evans, it takes recognition that all voices in the medical encounter have things to say that are as important as one's own statements. It takes listening aligned toward *understanding*, not just the collection of factual data. And it takes raising one's awareness to clues – nonverbal signals, fleeting glimpses of emotion, and key words (such as worried, concerned, and afraid) – and following up on these clues when they present themselves.[53,54] The essence of ensemble, whether in jazz or in medicine, lies in looking beyond one's own perspective to see, understand, and respond to the perspectives of others.

Coda

The improvisational concepts of space, voice, and ensemble all go beyond a prevailing understanding of communication as verbal information exchange, and they foster a more holistic and contextualized view of communicative phenomena.[55] For example, the concept of improvisational voice provides a bridge between basic communication skills training and the complexity of communication in real-world settings, because it provides a conceptual frame for viewing the integrated performance of multiple communication skills and patterns. Voice suggests that, beyond developing and demonstrating proficiency in individual skills, learners must also begin to develop their own personal style in applying those skills. This process raises some important questions for future work: How can one assess the progress of learners' development of their own unique voice? Does the development of voice occur in discrete stages or along a continuum? What kinds of activities (e.g., reflection, observation with feedback) or combinations of activities foster physicians' development of voice? In what ways might the traditions of jazz education be applied in medical communication skills training? How does the development of voice relate to patient-centered outcomes, such as trust, participation, and satisfaction? If physicians bring their unique voice to the medical encounter, how would that relate to physician satisfaction and the prevention of burnout? In a similar fashion, the jazz concepts of space and ensemble may also lead to new directions for education and research.

In today's world of evidence and guidelines, physicians are at risk for reducing patients' complex diagnoses to simple algorithms that do not take into account critical contextual information.[13] This risk exists as well for patient-physician communication. Physicians who focus on only a fixed set of questions or follow the same sequence of inquiry for every patient will miss opportunities to hear the patient's perspective, build partnerships, and bring their own selves to the work of patient care. Physicians must be skilled improvisers, able to efficiently explore the unique aspects of a patient's illness and communicate in a way that is in harmony with that patient's style, all while managing the tension between new territory and the established patterns inherent in their communicative and clinical training. As educators and researchers, we can draw on the traditions and knowledge of jazz musicians as we try to enhance the quality of improvisation in the medical encounter.

The real power and innovation of jazz is that a group of people can come together and create art – improvised art – and can negotiate their agendas with each other. And that negotiation is the art.

—Trumpeter Wynton Marsalis[20]

References

1. Stephenson S. Jazzed about Roy Haynes. *Smithsonian*. 2003; 34: 107–14.
2. McCroskey J, Richmond V. *Fundamentals of Human Communication: An Interpersonal Perspective*. Long Grove, Ill: Waveland Press; 1995.
3. Simpson M, Buckman R, Stewart M, et al. Doctor-patient communication: the Toronto consensus statement. *BMJ*. 1991; 303(6814): 1385–87.
4. Kohn L, Corrigan J, Donaldson M, eds. *To Err Is Human: Building a Safer Health System*. Washington, DC: National Academy Press; 2000.
5. Kaplan SH, Greenfield S, Ware JE Jr. Assessing the effects of physician-patient interactions on the outcomes of chronic disease. *Med Care*. 1989; 27(Suppl 3): S110–27.
6. Greenfield S, Kaplan S, Ware JE Jr. Expanding patient involvement in care. Effects on patient outcomes. *Ann Intern Med*. 1985; 102(4): 520–28.
7. Predictors of outcome in headache patients presenting to family physicians – a one year prospective study. The Headache Study Group of The University of Western Ontario. *Headache*. 1986; 26(6): 285–94.
8. Deyo RA, Diehl AK. Patient satisfaction with medical care for low-back pain. *Spine*. 1986; 11(1): 28–30.
9. Bartlett EE, Grayson M, Barker R, et al. The effects of physician communications skills on patient satisfaction; recall, and adherence. *J Chronic Dis*. 1984; 37(910): 755–64.
10. Levinson W, Roter DL, Mullooly JP, Dull VT, Frankel RM. Physician-patient communication. The relationship with malpractice claims among primary care physicians and surgeons. *JAMA*. 1997; 277(7): 553–59.
11. Ong LM, de Haes JC, Hoos AM, Lammes FB. Doctor-patient communication: a review of the literature. *Soc Sci Med*. 1995; 40(7): 903–18.
12. Hall JA, Roter DL, Katz NR. Meta-analysis of correlates of provider behavior in medical encounters. *Med Care*. 1988; 26(7): 657–75.
13. Shaughnessy AF, Slawson DC, Becker L. Clinical jazz: harmonizing clinical experience and evidence-based medicine. *J Fam Pract*. 1998; 47(6): 425–28.
14. Roter DL, Stewart M, Putnam SM, et al. Communication patterns of primary care physicians. *JAMA*. 1997; 277(4): 350–56.
15. Committee on Quality of Health Care in America, Institute of Medicine. *Crossing the Quality Chasm: A New Health System for the 21st Century*. Washington, DC: National Academy Press; 2001.
16. Kleinman A. *The Illness Narratives: Suffering, Healing and the Human Condition*. New York, NY: Basic Books; 1988.
17. Nachmanovitch S. *Free Play: Improvisation in Life and Art*. New York, NY: Tarcher/Putnam; 1990.
18. Miller WL, McDaniel RR Jr, Crabtree BF, Stange KC. Practice jazz: understanding variation in family practices using complexity science. *J Fam Pract*. 2001; 50(10): 872–78.

19. Barrett FJ. Creativity and improvisation in jazz and organizations: implications for organizational learning. *Org Sci*. 1998; 9: 88–105.
20. Ward G, Burns K. *Jazz: A History of America's Music*. New York, NY: Knopf/Random House; 2000.
21. King J. *What Jazz Is: An Insider's Guide to Understanding and Listening to Jazz*. New York, NY: Walker; 1997.
22. Nisenson E. *Round About Midnight: A Portrait of Miles Davis*. New York, NY: Da Capo Press; 1996.
23. Roter D, Hall J. *Doctors Talking With Patients/Patients Talking With Doctors*. Westport, Conn: Auburn House; 1993.
24. Roter DL, Larson S, Shinitzky H, et al. Use of an innovative video feedback technique to enhance communication skills training. *Med Educ*. 2004; 38(2): 145–57.
25. Stiles WB, Putnam SM. Verbal exchanges in medical interviews: concepts and measurement. *Soc Sci Med*. 1992; 35(3): 347–55.
26. Inui TS, Carter WB, Kukull WA, Haigh VH. Outcome-based doctor-patient interaction analysis: I. Comparison of techniques. *Med Care*. 1982; 20(6): 535–49.
27. Del Piccolo L, Putnam SM, Mazzi MA, Zimmermann C. The biopsychosocial domains and the functions of the medical interview in primary care: construct validity of the Verona Medical Interview Classification System. *Patient Educ Couns*. 2004; 53(1): 47–56.
28. Barr DA. A time to listen. *Ann Intern Med*. 2004; 140(2): 144.
29. Hentoff N. Untitled liner notes from the CD *The Legendary OKEH and Epic Recordings by Ahmad Jamal*. Epic/Legacy Recordings; 2005.
30. Haidet P, Paterniti DA. "Building" a history rather than "taking" one: a perspective on information sharing during the medical interview. *Arch Intern Med*. 2003; 163(10): 1134–40.
31. Frankel RM, Stein T. Getting the most out of the clinical encounter: the four habits model. *J Med Pract Manage*. 2001; 16(4): 184–91.
32. Kleinman AM. Interpreting illness meanings: the clinician's mini-ethnography. *Med Encounter*. 1986; 3: 5–7.
33. Marvel MK, Epstein RM, Flowers K, Beckman HB. Soliciting the patient's agenda: have we improved? *JAMA*. 1999; 281(3): 283–87.
34. Frankel RM, Beckman HB. The pause that refreshes. *Hosp Pract (Off Ed)*. 1988; 23(9A): 62, 65–67.
35. Beckman H, Frankel R. The impact of physician behavior on the collection of data. *Ann Intern Med*. 1984; 101: 692–96.
36. Ellison R. *Living With Music: Ralph Ellison's Jazz Writings*. New York, NY: The Modern Library; 2002.
37. Epstein RM. Mindful practice. *JAMA*. 1999; 282(9): 833–39.
38. Novack DH, Suchman AL, Clark W, Epstein RM, Najberg E, Kaplan C. Calibrating the physician. Personal awareness and effective patient care. Working Group on Promoting Physician Personal Awareness, American Academy on Physician and Patient. *JAMA*. 1997; 278(6): 502–09.
39. Nisenson E. *Ascension: John Coltrane and His Quest*. New York, NY: Da Capo Press; 1995.
40. Smith R. *The Patient's Story: Integrated Patient-Doctor Interviewing*. Boston, Mass: Little Brown; 1996.
41. Coulehan J, Block M. *The Medical Interview: Mastering Skills for Clinical Practice*. 3rd ed. Philadelphia, Pa: FA Davis; 1997.
42. Quill TE, Townsend P. Bad news: delivery, dialogue, and dilemmas. *Arch Intern Med*. 1991; 151(3): 463–68.
43. Baile WF, Buckman R, Lenzi R, et al. SPIKES – A six-step protocol for delivering bad news: application to the patient with cancer. *Oncologist*. 2000; 5(4): 302–11.
44. Garg A, Buckman R, Kason Y. Teaching medical students how to break bad news. *CMAJ*. 1997; 156(8): 1159–64.

45. Beach MC, Inui T. Relationship-centered care. A constructive reframing. *J Gen Intern Med.* 2006; 21(Suppl 1): S3–S8.
46. Evans B. Improvisation in Jazz. Liner notes from the CD *Kind of Blue* by Miles Davis: Columbia/Legacy; 1997.
47. Pettinger P. *Bill Evans: How My Heart Sings.* New Haven, Conn: Yale University Press; 2002.
48. Street R. Accommodation in medical consultations. In: Giles H, Coupland N, Coupland J, eds. *Contexts of Accommodation: Developments in Applied Sociolinguistics.* Cambridge, Mass: Cambridge University Press; 1991.
49. Platt FW, McMath JC. Clinical hypocompetence: the interview. *Ann Intern Med.* 1979; 91(6): 898–902.
50. Platt FW, Platt CM. Two collaborating artists produce a work of art: the medical interview. *Arch Intern Med.* 2003; 163(10): 1131–32.
51. Kleinman A, Eisenberg L, Good B. Culture, illness, and care: clinical lessons from anthropologic and cross-cultural research. *Ann Intern Med.* 1978; 88(2): 251–58.
52. Heisler M, Vijan S, Anderson RM, et al. When do patients and their physicians agree on diabetes treatment goals and strategies, and what difference does it make? *J Gen Intern Med.* 2003; 18(11): 893–902.
53. Levinson W, Gorawara-Bhat R, Lamb J. A study of patient clues and physician responses in primary care and surgical settings. *JAMA.* 2000; 284(8): 1021–27.
54. Lang F, Floyd MR, Beine KL. Clues to patients' explanations and concerns about their illnesses. A call for active listening. *Arch Fam Med.* 2000; 9(3): 222–27.
55. Haidet P. Finding our way 'into the pocket' with patients. *Med Encounter.* 2005; 19(2): 34.

22

Gazing at the Future

Steve M. Blevins, MD

JERRY NEVER COMPLAINS. HE IS 58 YEARS OLD AND INSEPARABLE FROM his wife, Betty. They are irrepressibly cheerful – synesthetic, in fact: when one laughs, the other cheers. As teenagers, they fell in love, and in love they remain. They are masters of resilience – emotionally, that is. Physically, Jerry has struggled, but he is better now because of Betty and ready for a 40th "honeymoon." Soon they will be sunbathing in the Caribbean.

I am delighted to see Jerry and Betty at the end of a long day. Jerry is sitting on the examination table, quiet and motionless. He has lost a few pounds but is still plump. His thin, straw hair is neatly cut. His brown eyes are magnified by thick lenses. He looks awkward in an undersized gown. Staring ahead, he seems transfixed by the empty wall before him. Betty stands by him, her arm draped casually around his shoulder.

"Good afternoon," I say.

"Hi, Dr Blevins," they reply.

I smile at Betty and turn to Jerry.

"So, Jerry, where are you taking your lovely bride?"

He grins and glances at his wife. "Anguilla," he mumbles.

"Really?" I ask. "Why Anguilla?"

His face brightens; his eyes sparkle. He begins to rhapsodize on the charms of Anguilla, or so I suppose, for I cannot understand a word he is saying. Still, his enthusiasm is unmistakable.

Betty understands every word. She translates: "Anguilla has sun-drenched beaches, pristine waters, and midnight barbecue." Then realizing that she sounds like a brochure, she laughs and adds, "Jerry's dreaming of the barbecue. I'm dreaming of the beach."

Jerry is amused, which brings joy to his wife.

"Are you healthy enough to go, Jerry?" I ask teasingly.

"You bet!" he mumbles.

I look at Betty, as if needing confirmation. "Is he telling the truth?"

"He certainly is," she replies. "He's having a little trouble with balance, but he walks every day."

Jerry's tremors began when he was 30 years old. Two years later, Parkinson's disease was diagnosed. His condition has progressed slowly. Last year, he received a brain stimulator, which he loves. His tremors are gone now, but his voice is muffled and his limbs are stiff. He cannot write, but he can walk alone, although he prefers to hold Betty's hand.

Pulling out my stethoscope, I check his blood pressure and examine him. As always, I regale him with stories of my weekend adventures. He enjoys my stories, even the silly ones.

"Well, everything checks out," I conclude. "You're good to go! Have a safe trip and don't eat too much."

I leave the room smiling. Jerry and Betty have a magical effect on me. Their joy is contagious.

Returning to my office, I sit at my desk and dictate a few notes. After completing my work, I reach into the top drawer, pull out a bottle, and remove a large orange pill. With a swig of water, I swallow the day's last dose of levodopa.

Leaning back in my chair, I reflect on the events of last spring: the first time my hand fumbled while combing my hair, the morning I first used two hands to brush my teeth, the afternoon I began to have trouble writing.

I was 45 years old and I was convinced that I had injured my arm at the gym. When my condition did not improve, I arranged to see my doctor.

I remember his kindness. He listened carefully to my story and tested my arm in a dozen ways. His examination ended with an apocalyptic request: he asked me to tap my feet. The request seemed superfluous, because I could run and swim without difficulty. I acquiesced, and to my astonishment, my right foot faltered.

My journey into the surreal may have lasted only a second. I heard children giggling in a distant examination room and smelled alcohol from the adjacent sink. I noticed a cricket in the overhead light and saw patches of light and dark on my doctor's white coat.

My disease was nameless, but I knew the essentials: It was central, neurological, and surely progressive. When the name Parkinson's was introduced, the mystery had already lost its sting.

For several days I was too distracted to work. I barely listened to my patients and wrote the wrong date on prescriptions. Impatiently I waited for the weekend with its promise of isolation. When Friday arrived, I was too preoccupied to notice Jerry's arrival.

Dazed, I entered the room and looked at him. He was perched comfortably on the examination table. Betty stood quietly beside him. Perhaps we conversed. One memory remains: As I approached him with my stethoscope, we looked at each other – he with his Parkinsonian stare; I with the gaze of abject fear. I imagined his decades-long struggle: the frozen movements, the shaking, the distorted voice, the stimulator. He was a crystal ball through which I saw my own bleak future. I wondered when my movements would congeal, when my voice would fade, when …

Jerry's smile interrupted my reverie. I began to examine him. I checked his blood pressure and listened to his heart, but I could only think of his silent immobility.

As I listened to his lungs, he began to snicker. Sometimes Jerry behaved oddly. I usually delighted in his eccentricity, but not today. I was in no mood for his antics. From the corner of my eye I could see Betty's nervous expression. Raising her finger to her mouth, she encouraged her husband to shush. But Jerry kept smiling.

"What is it, Jerry?" I asked.

He turned to Betty and mumbled something, but perturbed, she ignored his childish behavior. Jerry waited for the translation, knowing that Betty would eventually give in. Soon her expression softened, and with rolling eyes, she said, "Dr Blevins, Jerry wants you to know that you have shaving cream in your ear."

That evening I sat on my bed and looked out the window. The park was lovely with its vernal backdrop of blue skies and green fields. An old man was riding a bicycle. A mother was pushing a baby carriage. Children were racing on their skateboards.

I thought about Jerry. His happiness defied nature; it was perennial. For 10 years I had reveled in his good humor, though now it seemed eerie and discordant. My despair, of course, seemed justified – but why? My limitations were few and mild. Jerry, by contrast, was almost mute, but seemed oblivious to his condition. Was he unrealistic? Was I?

Spring drifted into summer, and Jerry returned to clinic with his usual cheer. During his visit, I glanced at him repeatedly, hoping to glimpse the future. His condition had not changed: His eyes were unblinking; his pose was statuesque. But the crystal ball, which penetrated deeper, revealed a future less foreboding. His suffering, though still extant, was subsumed by a graceful serenity. Perhaps I had misread the future last spring. Perhaps time had sharpened my foresight.

I thought about Jerry throughout the summer.

Then one day Betty called to say that Jerry wanted to go to the Caribbean. They had never been there, and with their 40th anniversary approaching, they were determined to go. Jerry needed a "preflight clearance" and had scheduled an appointment to see me.

And so he arrives today, fit to travel. His blood pressure is normal. His neurological condition, though advanced, is safely quarantined from his happy life. He has heard the Caribbean's call and will pursue its promise of sunny beaches and midnight barbecue.

Daylight has passed along with my daydream. The clinic is empty. I put on my coat and turn out the light. For a moment I imagine Jerry in a swimsuit, covered head-to-toe in sunscreen, mumbling and fumbling on the beach. Maybe it is time to stop thinking about the future. After all, there is no crystal ball, just a mirror reflecting the obvious: Jerry is happy.

And I am happy thinking of Jerry dreaming of Anguilla.

Section 5

Knowledge

Ian McWhinney, a pioneer of family medicine, once described his specialty as "the product of a ferment of ideas. To understand family medicine, therefore, it is necessary to have a grasp of the ideas on which medicine is based. Moreover, it is important for a newly emergent discipline to be based on firm theoretical foundations."[1]

Although no longer newly emergent, family medicine in the United States continues to evolve and re-form as it strives to meet the challenges of an unsustainable health care system. In this process of reinvention, "the ferment of ideas" remains vitally important. To help create a health care system that values quality, relationship-centered care,[2] primary care specialties must know who they are. To discover new paths in patient care and policy, they must know where they've been. To create ideas that are fresh and forward-looking, they must understand the concepts that have guided them so far.

The articles in this section delve into the following concepts fundamental to understanding family medicine and primary care.

- *Theory*: Paul Thomas elucidates the theories of knowledge that underscore three basic functions of primary care: listening, reflecting, and diagnosing. Understanding these theories, he posits, will help demystify the core of generalist practice.
- *Evidence*: should clinical decisions be based on evidence or experience? Zachary Flake, a self-described member of "the evidence-based generation," shares his struggle to balance information, intuition, and compassion.
- *Training*: James Glazer recalls the first time, as a family medicine trainee, he saw a beating heart. Unlike popular portrayals of medical miracles, the

experience was characterized by moral quandary, emergency room chaos, and sweat.

- *Leadership*: Ian Douglas Couper considers how feeling important stifles leadership. True leadership depends on teamwork, openness, and self-reflection.
- *Community engagement*: if efforts to improve community health are to succeed, community members must be heard. Andrew Sussman and Marino Rivera recount the experience of a researcher who was welcomed into a mountain village, but only after listening deeply and absorbing the cultural wisdom of a local resident.
- *Reflection*: one night in the Israeli desert, Jeffrey Borkan tried, unsuccessfully, to revive a car crash victim – a young, newly wed woman. This story is moving in its own right and exemplifies the depth and meaning that can be found in medical narrative.
- *Writing*: the act of writing helps us create, think, and heal. How, though, do busy professionals find time to write? Lucy Candib offers three real-life strategies.

References

1. McWhinney IR. *An Introduction to Family Medicine*. New York, NY: Oxford University Press; 1981. p. 23.
2. Roberts RG, Snape PS, Burke K. Task Force Report 5. Report of the Task Force on Family Medicine's Role in Shaping the Future Health Care Delivery System. *Ann Fam Med*. 2004; 2(Suppl 1): S88–99.

23

General Medical Practitioners Need to Be Aware of the Theories on Which Our Work Depends

Paul Thomas, FRCGP, MD

Introduction

Good general medical practice should be based on evidence whenever appropriate and possible, but what form of evidence can do justice to the multifaceted world I encounter as a general practitioner/family physician? First, I share with specialists a need for objective evidence about harm to patients from known conditions – asthma, bed-wetting, cancer, debt (and all conditions beginning with the other letters of the alphabet). Second, I need to generate evidence about hidden and interconnected things in patients' lives, such as loss of purpose or relationship difficulties. Finally, I need to bring together a diversity of objective and subjective evidence to develop with a patient a unique plan that will improve more than one thing at the same time.

Evidence is knowledge generated from competent inquiry. Evidence, however, is commonly associated with a particular approach to inquiry called *positivism* (quantitative research). Inquiry helps me with the first of my three needs when I need objective evidence about known diseases in simple, controlled situations. It is less reliable, however, in complex and changing situations.[1-3]

An image that reveals the limitations of positivism is a game of billiards. Each ball has weight and shape that does not change during the game. When one ball hits another, it causes movement that is predictable because everything else stays still, which is the definition of a controlled laboratory. The world experienced by general medical practitioners, however, often lacks such simplicity and predictability. Patients, unlike billiard balls, are undergoing constant change internally, and externally so are their contexts (relationships, jobs, organizations, projects). Consider the complexity of the task that would face a billiard player if the properties and trajectories of the balls and the table were all changing simultaneously.

Simplicity and predictability do not make positivism wrong; they merely limit it. On its own, positivism can lead to overly simplistic ideas that prevent us from realizing our potential to heal or harm people. To understand what generalists must do in less straightforward situations, we must develop an approach that goes beyond positivistic assumptions about the world.

In this essay I wish to argue that the complex, uncertain, and creative aspects of the role of a generalist medical practitioner can be understood by complementing positivist theory of knowledge with two other respected and equally important theories termed *critical theory* and *constructivism*.[4] Using all three theories in clinical practice requires complementing diagnosing with listening and reflection. In research and audit it requires complementing quantitative inquiry with exploratory and participatory approaches.

I want to go further. I want to argue that you will already know and practice these approaches, but you may lack the language to talk about it and consequently be held back from improving your skills. In the English-speaking world philosophy is rarely part of a medical student curriculum. As a result, theory of knowledge is considered by many to be irrelevant. I want to argue the opposite – it provides language to explain the essence of generalist practice that is usually described as a mystery.[5]

Positivism, Critical Theory, and Constructivism

To distinguish their unique features, I describe in this section the assumptions made by positivism, critical theory, and constructivism about the nature of reality and the generation of knowledge. I then argue that each of these three approaches offers equal but different insights into the complex evolving stories that patients tell us. Finally, I suggest how general medical practice can improve its use of all three theories in combination.

Positivism

Positivism expects the world to be ordered simply and to be predictable. Entities really exist, unchanging and irrespective of other things. This assumption is called a critical realist ontology[4] (Table 1 displays definitions of ontology, epistemology, and methodology. The word *critical* distinguishes postpositivism from traditional positivism that held the naïve view that what was seen was the whole truth. Postpositivists accept that the world is more complex than superficial insights reveal.) Truth is like a nugget of gold waiting to be recognized. I know it is there because tests detect its objective presence (its epistemology is dualist-objectivist). Its methodology is experimental-manipulative – "a question or hypothesis is stated in advance in propositional form and subjected to empirical tests under control-led conditions."[4] This approach uses research methods, such as experiments, in which features of interest are named in advance, measured, and counted. Validity requires a statistical difference between these numbers. This theory has no power to reveal context (discrete features are counted in isolation from other things), and no power to reveal novelty (things must be named in advance).

TABLE 1 Definitions of ontology, epistemology, and methodology

Ontology	Ontology is concerned with the assumptions made by different beliefs about reality.[4,6] I am asking an ontological question when I ask, "In what ways is something really there?" If I believe that a stone has a discrete, enduring existence separate from everything else, and a smile has a transient existence that marks a meaningful transaction between people, I am making an ontological distinction.
Epistemology	Epistemology seeks to define knowledge within a particular belief about reality.[6,7] I am asking an epistemological question when I ask, "What is the relationship between the knower and the known?"[4] If I believe that a patient can subjectively experience the effect of a drug differently from a claim made by scientific evidence, I am making an epistemological distinction.
Methodology	Methodology is the study of ways of knowing within a particular belief about reality.[6] I am asking a methodological question when I ask, "What approach to knowledge generation will provide a reliable answer to my question?" I make different methodological choices when I invite respondents to (1) score a pick-list of options, (2) speak in their own words, or (3) participate in a focus group.

The French philosopher Auguste Comte coined the term positivism in the 19th century. It was a reaction against the theological and metaphysical understand-ings of knowledge that predated it. These previous understandings considered that truth was too complex and interconnected to be understood by mere mortals – personal struggle and contemplation guided by priests would reveal the best next steps in a world that was ultimately unknowable.

The new science was empowering, allowing people to predict what would happen in simple situations. For example, travelers can trust the structural integrity of airplanes, and doctors can know what forms of treatment are better at curing named diseases. The weakness of this type of knowledge is that it cannot reliably interpret interdependent and coevolving phenomena.

Take the example of depression. Although evidence from positivist inquiry helps me to recognize the features of depression and consider a range of reliable treatment options, as a generalist, I know that depression is not one entity. It is a feeling that arises from multiple coincidental and interacting factors. Inside depression can be found personal inadequacy, unresolved past hurts, physical disease, bullying at work, genetic predisposition, dysfunctional families, and many other things, all compounding and causing each other. By helping patients to bring into view the range of factors that contribute to their depression, I can help them to help themselves. When I help patients in this way, they often say as they leave: "You know – I feel better just from having come."

When I explore these issues with a patient, I am considering the diagnosis of depression, not as the end of the matter, but the start of an exploration of something complex. Multiple factors are constantly affecting each other and adapting to changes in each other. The best plan includes a set of complementary actions to reduce harm and increase healthy ones. Positivism obstructs this exploration of complexity because it reduces rather than expands the horizon of inquiry. This reductionist tendency of positivism provoked researchers to develop exploratory and participatory approaches to inquiry that became known as qualitative research. Qualitative research was originally defined as anything that was not quantitative (positivist). In time researchers came to agree that qualitative research includes both critical theory and constructivism, which together can generate knowledge about contexts and innovation that are invisible to positivism.

Critical Theory

The theory of knowledge that best reveals the context of a phenomenon is called critical (social) theory or "ideologically oriented inquiry."[4] As with positivism its ontology is critical realist – truth is still expected to be really there but hidden by more superficial or transient truths. The researcher considers different perspectives and meanings that are not immediately obvious. Its epistemology is subjectivist in that critical theory values what people know from experience. Its methodology is dialogic – people of different perspectives debate the rights and wrongs of different versions of the truth to remove false consciousness and arrive at a better version of the truth. This approach uses research methods, such as case studies that "focus on a contemporary phenomenon within some real-life context."[7] Validity requires concordance between different perceptions (termed *triangulation*) that pinpoints the so-called real truth.

The origins of critical theory are attributed to the German philosopher Jurgen Habermas, who maintained that our understandings of the world are distorted because we are blind to much of what is relevant.[8] Contemporary application of critical theory is "concerned in particular with issues of power and justice and the ways that the economy, matters of race, class and gender, ideologies, discourses, education, religion and other social institutions, and cultural dynamics interact to construct a social system."[9]

Constructivism

Novelty and innovation are best understood through the theory of knowledge termed *constructivism*,[4] associated with the concept of social constructionism.[10] Constructivism maintains that truth is a coconstructed phenomenon – "findings are literally the creation of the process of interaction between the inquirer and the inquired … who become fused into a single (monist) entity."[4] For example, gravity is a manifestation of the attractive properties of matter; love is a manifestation of shared meaning between two people. These interactions have, not a realist, but a relativist ontology[4] – true-to-those-involved. The ontological-epistemological distinction is obliterated in constructivism, because what is really there and the relation of the observer-participant to it are different versions of the same question. This approach uses such research methods as appreciative inquiry[11] and participatory action research,[12] which facilitate mutual learning, emergent understandings, and consensus. Validity requires that seemingly contradictory things make sense as a whole to the persons involved (termed *crystallization of meaning*).[13]

Constructivism reveals the cocreative nature of innovation. A genuinely new insight, by definition, has not yet been formed. Instead, it emerges through complex responsive processes.[14] The result is not the property of one or another author, but a shared entwining that also has its own unique identity and properties. The idea of a photograph and the idea of radio waves both contributed to the idea of television. Two parents give life to a child. It may be possible to track connections between new and old, but the television and the child are different from the things that gave them birth and are genuinely new.

Positivism, Critical Theory, and Constructivism Provide Complementary Insights into Stories in Evolution

I am putting forward the idea that theories are not truth as such but are lenses that filter certain elements from complex wholes. This concept is not new. As Heisenberg said: "What we observe is not nature itself, but nature exposed to our method of questioning."[15] Different kinds of lenses or questions produce different kinds of truth or answers.

This type of filtering is what happens when we use our senses to "see" a garden. When I "look" at it with my ears, I hear bird song. If I "look" with my nose, I smell flower pollen. My eyes see colorful trees and bushes. My different senses filter from the fuller picture those aspects that resonate with the way I am looking.

I can look at a garden using the eyes of the three theories of knowledge described above. If I look with the eyes of positivism, I see what can be named and counted – birdsong, scent, and trees. If I look with the eyes of critical theory, I can see more hidden or interconnected truths – the effect of wind and the changing seasons on plant growth. If I look with the eyes of constructivism, I will see processes of creative interaction – bees pollinating flowers and birds building nests from whatever materials are available. Each insight is valuable, but none captures it all. Together the insights reveal a fuller, moving picture. The responsibility is mine to discern what meaning it has for me as a whole.

We also use these three theories when making decisions about how to act. When a bus is speeding toward me, I quickly jump out of the way, making a positivist prediction that the bus will harm me. When I wish to make a complicated journey, however, I will search the timetables of buses and trains for routes that were invisible at first sight to me (critical theory). During the journey I may change my mind about my destination as I experience the difficulties in getting there and the attractiveness of other opportunities that have opened up for me (constructivism).

Complexity theorists call these three theories simple, complicated, and complex. In complicated situations the best option must be puzzled out more than in simple ones, but a correct solution will still be waiting to be discovered. By contrast, complexity "arises from the interaction between the components of a system and its environment."[16] Answers do not preexist and must be created through multiple adaptations of the related components.[17]

In general practice we often encounter complexity, for example when someone has several complaints. The best way forward involves lateral thinking (a combination of critical theory and constructivism). Evidence from the past (re-search

= searching again) contributes only in part to this forward-looking process (development = growth or evolution). Kierkegaard reminds us that many people inappropriately conflate research and development. He said: "Most organizational theorists, as well as most philosophers, mistake the certainty of structures seen in hindsight for the emergent order that frames living forward. Neither group of scholars has come to grips with the fact that their conceptual understandings trail life and are of a different character than is living forward."[18]

Evidence carries with it an imprint of the context of its generation. We cannot assume that evidence will be meaningful in other contexts and to those who do not share that context. Evidence should be food for thought rather than an authority that cannot be challenged – evidence is a snapshot of more-complex stories-in-evolution.

It is within stories that different kinds of evidence can be integrated. Each person thinks of his or her life as an integrated whole story – what MacIntyre calls narrative unity.[19] Communities likewise wish to share a coherent history. In health the integrity of the whole story is maintained. Diseases can challenge this integrity. Evidence must illuminate both.

Implications for Generalist Medical Practice

We consciously or unconsciously use these three theories of knowledge in the consulting room when diagnosing, listening, and reflecting:

When I have reason to consider meningitis, positivism is my dominant approach. I take care to identify the characteristic features. Conversely, when trying to understand how multiple illnesses affect someone, I will use open questions (as in critical theory) to listen to what the patient has to say. When there are many possible ways forward, I ask the patient to go away to reflect (as will I), agreeing to meet again to devise the best overall plan (constructivism).

When a patient has hypertension, I may review the scientific evidence (positivism), but then reason that the evidence is based on a study with subjects younger than the person in front of me; it may therefore not be relevant in this context, and I may accept a different blood pressure than the evidence suggests (critical theory). I may then ask what the patient's preferences and practical constraints are, devising a personalized plan (constructivism).

Knowing the three different kinds of knowledge helps me to be a better clinician. Rather than listening merely to detect signs of a particular diagnosis, critical theory leads me to hear what someone is struggling to say in his or her own terms. Constructivism leads me to reflect ideas and experiences against others (the meaning of the word *reflection*), searching for interesting connections. From this playful interaction emerge new ways forward that no one had considered at the outset.

Knowing the three different kinds of knowledge helps me as a researcher to use qualitative inquiry, first as a prelude to finding the best thing to measure, and then as a way to reveal the complex interconnections within seemingly simple situations. It reminds me to facilitate participation in research and audit by stakeholders in care pathways[20] and whole systems,[21] not merely to facilitate later compliance, but also to generate the most trustworthy evidence for that context. There are many examples of how these three approaches produce competent practitioners and managers as well as better primary health care.[22]

We can contribute to the advancement of these ideas by supporting the following stances:

A narrative-based approach to consulting can lead to patients thinking differently about their lives, which will improve their overall health.[23] Listening and reflection in the consulting room should reinforce a practitioner's interpretations and facilitate a "meeting between experts,"[24] wherein each listens and shares perspectives, negotiating what should and should not require medical treatment.

A multimethod, transdisciplinary, participatory approach to research and audit should replace the current unbalanced focus on quantitative inquiries.[25] We should encourage complex interventions[26] that allow patients to tell their own stories,[27] and participatory inquiry[28,29] that builds learning communities.[30]

Learning and change are complex, multileveled activities that go beyond the learning of facts.[31] A learning organization[32] uses these three theories of knowledge by engaging in single-loop learning (positivism) that checks for errors, double-loop learning that reveals hidden forces (critical theory), and deutero-learning that generates new understandings from team learning (constructivism).[31]

References

1. Rosser WW. Application of evidence from randomised controlled trials to general practice. *Lancet*. 1999; 353: 661–64.
2. Rothwell PM. External validity of randomised controlled trials: "to whom do the results of this trial apply?" *Lancet*. 2005; 365: 82–93.
3. Griffiths F, Green E, Tsouroufli M. The nature of medical evidence and its inherent uncertainty for the clinical consultation: qualitative study. *BMJ*. 2005; 330: 511.
4. Guba E. *The Paradigm Dialog*. Newbury Park, CA: Sage Publications; 1990.
5. Heath I. *The Mystery of General Practice*. London: Nuffield Provincial Hospitals Trust; 1995.

6. Crabtree B, Miller W. Clinical research: a multimethod typology and qualitative roadmap. In: Crabtree B, Miller W, eds. *Doing Qualitative Research*. Thousand Oaks, CA: Sage Publications; 1999: 3–30.

7. Yin RK. *Case Study Research*. Thousand Oaks, CA: Sage Publications; 1994.

8. Wulff H, Pederson A, Rosenburg R. *Philosophy of Medicine: An Introduction*. Oxford: Blackwell; 1990.

9. Kincheloe JL, McLaren P. Rethinking critical theory and qualitative research. In: Denzin N, Lincoln Y, eds. *Handbook of Qualitative Research*. Thousand Oaks, CA: Sage Publications; 2000. Chapter 10.

10. Shotter J. *Conversational Realities: Constructing Life Through Language*. London: Sage Publications; 2000.

11. Whitney D, Trosten-Bloom A. *The Power of Appreciative Inquiry*. San Francisco, CA: Berrett-Koehler; 2003.

12. Whyte WF. *Participatory Action Research*. New York, NY: Sage Publications; 1991.

13. Janesick VJ. The choreography of qualitative research design. In: Denzin N, Lincoln Y, eds. *Handbook of Qualitative Research*. Thousand Oaks, CA: Sage Publications; 2000. Chapter 13.

14. Stacey R. *Complex Responsive Processes in Organizations*. London: Routledge; 2001.

15. Capra F. *The Web of Life*. London: Flamingo; 1997.

16. Hassey A. Complexity and the clinical encounter. In: Sweeney K, Griffiths F, eds. *Complexity and Healthcare: An Introduction*. Oxford: Radcliffe Medical Press; 2002. pp. 59–74.

17. Plsek P. Redesigning health care with insights from the science of complex adaptive systems. In: *Crossing the Quality Chasm: A New Health System for the 21st Century*. Hyattsville, Md: National Academy Press; 2000. pp. 309–22.

18. Weick KE. That's moving: theories that matter. *J Management Inq*. 1999; 8: 134–42.

19. MacIntyre A. *After Virtue*. London: Duckworth; 2000.

20. Thomas P, Oni L, Alli M, et al. Antenatal screening for haemoglobinopathies in primary care: a whole system participatory action research project. *Br J Gen Pract*. 2005; 55: 424–28.

21. Thomas P, McDonnell J, McCulloch J, et al. Increasing capacity for innovation in bureaucratic primary care organizations: a whole system participatory action research project. *Ann Fam Med*. 2005; 3: 312–17.

22. Thomas P. *Integrating Primary Health Care: Leading, Managing, Facilitating*. Oxford: Radcliffe Publishing; 2006.

23. Launer J. *Narrative-based Primary Care. A Practical Guide*. Oxford: Radcliffe Medical Press; 2002.

24. Tuckett D, Boulton M, Olson C, Williams A. *Meetings Between Experts*. London: Tavistock; 1985.

25. Stange KC, Miller WL, McWhinney I. Developing the knowledge base of family practice. *Fam Med*. 2001; 33: 286–97.

26. Campbell M, Fitzpatrick R, Haines A, et al. Framework for design and evaluation of complex interventions to improve health. *BMJ*. 2000; 321: 694–96.

27. Greenhalgh T, Collard A, Begum N. Sharing stories: complex intervention for diabetes education in minority ethnic groups who do not speak English. *BMJ*. 2005; 330: 628.

28. Macaulay AC, Commanda LE, Freeman WL, et al. Participatory research maximises community and lay involvement. North American Primary Care Research Group. *BMJ*. 1999; 319: 774–78.

29. Reason P. Three approaches to participative inquiry. In: Denzin N, Lincoln Y, eds. *Handbook of Qualitative Research*. Thousand Oaks, CA: Sage Publications; 1994. Chapter 20.

30. Wenger E. Communities of practice and social learning systems. *Organization*. 2000; 7: 225–46.

31. Argyris C, Schon DA. *Organizational Learning II: Theory, Method and Practice*. Boston, Mass: Addison Wesley; 1996.

32. Senge P. *The Fifth Discipline*. London: Century Hutchinson; 1993.

24

The Irreverent Nature of Evidence

Zachary Flake, MD

THE GRAYING INTERNIST STARED AT THE BOARD AND READIED HIS CHALK. So far, my case presentation at morning report had gone smoothly. Then, without a word, he held up his hand. I halted. He lowered his glasses and looked over the rims. "You transfused her? Even with her history of heart failure?"

"Yessir," I defended the decision. "She has symptomatic anemia."

"And how will you monitor for fluid overload?"

"I ordered a brain natriuretic peptide on admission and will repeat it tomorrow morning," I proposed.

"Ha!" he yelped and dropped his glasses on the table. "What ever happened to JVD and gallops and rales?"

I knew the correct response, but I couldn't verbalize it. Instead, I lowered my head and focused on the stack of papers before me. As I cowered, our family medicine attending physician, an outspoken woman trained in the era of evidence, came to my defense. "Let's face it," she reminded him, "the sensitivity and specificity of physical findings in congestive heart failure are terrible. The BNP is a much better way to follow fluid status."

The internist stepped back. We had ventured into statistics, and this was shaky ground. "I suppose you are correct," he conceded. He turned back to me. "What happened next?"

The debate over brain natriuretic peptide and many others like it are becoming increasingly common in hospitals and clinics across the country. They represent a surprising development in medicine during the last decade – the reliance on evidence to make decisions. This shift to evidence-based decision making is surprising because clinical practice hasn't been that way all along. When I entered medical school, I assumed (as many patients do) that decisions were based on studies, investigations, and trials. As I've watched my mentors and my colleagues throughout training, I've come to the remarkable conclusion that many physicians rely on something less quantitative but infinitely more visceral – experience. They teach with such statements as, "I know the studies say this … but one time I had that happen." Their experience-based practices are founded on common sense, but they are also sprinkled with isolated, frequently nonrepresentative, cases that cling to their memories because the cases are associated with the vivid emotions of being rebuked or even sued. More than I ever realized, medical decisions are human decisions, frequently based on instinct, personal interactions with a patient, and even how a doctor feels on a particular day.

Medical decisions will always be human ones, but the foundation for these judgments is changing. Mine is the evidence-based generation. We refuse to accept "because that has worked in the past" as justification for any decision. At the interface between experience and evidence, as in our morning report, conflict is frequent. We no longer learn exclusively from the experience of our mentors. When they offer an approach, we accept it cautiously. With this transition comes healthy questioning, sometimes even disrespect, about the source and the quality of information.

Lately I've been thinking this dispute is more than generational. Technology has forced us to reevaluate completely the role of information in medicine. As serious consumers, modern physicians must become evidence connoisseurs. My colleagues discuss the value of MDConsult, UpToDate, and InfoPOEMs, and we debate the usefulness of intention-to-treat analyses. When our mentors seek information, it is often derived from single sources and frequently based more on experience. We evaluate levels of evidence and scan for the most recent studies or meta-analyses. While the graying internist squints at the PDR, we tap away at our PDAs. Even so, we're all beginning to question how our reliance on evidence affects our relationships with patients.

It's hard for one generation of physicians to accept the approach of another. Older physicians lament the declining physical examination skills and loss of the art of medicine in their apprentices. Younger physicians deride older physicians as out-of-date and nostalgic. Older physicians rely on their central (as opposed to peripheral) brains to make point-of-care decisions and regard PDAs as crutches that can only soften the minds of younger physicians. Younger physicians have accepted that they cannot know everything, but that they must know how to find information quickly and evaluate its quality.

The Wonder and the Mystery

I suggest that the thoughtful family physician can learn something from both perspectives. The evidence-based approach certainly has something to offer – we realize that information mastery is no longer optional, it is a core requirement in a doctor's tool bag. We nimbly navigate an exponentially increasing library of medical evidence, and more than any generation in the past, we think in terms of efficiency and outcomes. We also tend to think in terms of machines and mechanics. All too often we view medicine from the outside, as huge groups of study participants viewed through various numbers and images.

Our experience-based advisors remind us that we have answered a noble and compassionate call. They personify an era when the doctor-patient relationship existed on a personal level with fewer distractions from laboratory tests and radiographs, an era when listening was a doctor's most effective skill. They come from a time when a study group was an N of 1 and doctors had a personal understanding of individual patients, and they use those understandings to make intuitive and intimate decisions. As we attempt to define our profession in this century, one of our greatest challenges is to remember the relationships that got us here. The mindful physician incorporates evidence and surveys outcomes, but never at the expense of a personal interaction with a patient.

In his essay "Leech, leech, et cetera," Lewis Thomas observes that modern clinicians have made a dangerous pact.[1] We crave technology and the information it provides, but in exchange we distance ourselves from patients and risk becoming simple technicians. The stethoscope, for example, magnifies visceral reverberations at the expense of a literal space between doctor and patient that did not exist before. Taken to the extreme, a radiologist can sit in his bedroom and use a CT scan to make a diagnosis that is more specific than the diagnosis of the bedside physician. Today, he notes, patients spend more time talking with the admissions and billing departments than with their doctor.

I'm trying not to let that happen to my patients. I paid attention to the BNP results, and I based my clinical decisions on them. I monitored the outcomes and prescribed medicines because they have improved morbidity and mortality in large studies. I've also come to realize that, whether he realized it or not, the graying internist was asking me not simply to look at my patient's neck and listen to her chest; he was urging me to be with my patient. When I look in the mirror some nights and see the technician that Thomas predicted, I wonder whether I might have something to learn from the internist after all.

Reference

1. Thomas L. Leech, leech, et cetera. In: *The Youngest Science: Notes of a Medicine-Watcher*. New York, NY: Penguin Books 1995.

25

Bag of Worms

James L. Glazer, MD, FACSM

"PUT YOUR HANDS IN THERE. BE CAREFUL NOT TO CUP YOUR FINGERS, though. Hold them out straight, like this," the surgeon told me and then demonstrated. "Squeeze gently, or else you'll puncture the myocardium." He looked me in the eye, "Have you ever done open cardiac massage before?" he asked.

I stared down in awe, shaking my head. Before me the patient's chest lay bared, the arcs of her ribs spread by the jaws of the retractor. Her pericardium, the fibrous sac covering her heart, was flayed open, and inside this gristly envelope the heart fibrillated. "Like a bag of worms," I thought, recalling the term from countless medical texts.

It had all begun for me 15 minutes earlier in the stairwell during another busy morning as a family medicine intern on the surgical service. I was minding my own business, walking upstairs to discharge Mr. Rossignol (name changed) to an alcohol rehabilitation facility when the hospital overhead pager squawked: "Respiratory to the ER STAT!" and a moment later, "Operating room crew to the ER STAT!" Clearly this was not the average emergency, so I aborted my ascent and galloped down the stairs.

The emergency department was a scene of pandemonium. A clump of personnel in baggy blue operating room scrubs spilled out of one of the rooms, revealing the site of the action. A drunk driver had struck a 28-year-old woman while she was on her way to pick up her infant from daycare. The driver of the other car was well known to us. His license had been revoked 3 times for driving under the influence. He frequented the wards of our hospital when his battered girlfriend refused to let him back inside her home. Today his luck had held; he was not seriously injured and lay across the hall on a stretcher, bellowing at the nurses to let him go home. One of them looked over to me and nodded at the intoxicated man. "You've heard the old saying," she said, "God looks after a drunk." She paused. "Too bad He doesn't also look after mothers," she added.

The woman had been conscious when the rescue squad found her, but she went into shock while the emergency crew extracted her from her mangled car. Her neck veins bulged as an ER physician intubated her. Then the surgeon snapped on his gloves and shouldered the nurses out of the way. He glanced up at me. "Come here," he said.

We painted her chest with sterile solution as the monitor showed her heartbeat slipping into dangerous arrhythmias and then back to normal again. Her fingers turned blue, then ashy gray, from lack of oxygen despite the anesthesiologist's efforts with the bag ventilator. "Hurry up if you want to help her," the surgeon prodded me.

I took an enormous cardiac needle from its plastic sheath, hoping that my movements would disguise the shaking of my hands. It looked impossibly long, like a prop from a Frankenstein movie. I stopped with the needle poised over her chest and looked up. The surgeon nodded to me.

The sensation of driving the needle through the layers of her chest wall was strange. The tissues seemed to adhere to the shaft as I haltingly advanced until I felt a soft pop. Suddenly the syringe blossomed with dark crimson blood. The surgeon nudged me and pointed at the monitor. While we watched, it traced the familiar pattern of a normal sinus rhythm. Relieving the pressure of the accumulated blood around the heart allowed it to beat normally again. As I moved away, I stumbled. In my tension I had been clenching my toes inside my shoes the whole time.

The patient's recovery was short-lived, and she soon slipped back into ventricular fibrillation. The cardiac needle clotted, and the surgeon called for the chest tray. With the ambulance lights flashing in our faces, the surgeon opened her chest. Using quick, confident strokes, he drew the scalpel blade over her ribs and bared the creamy yellow fat beneath the surface of her skin. Her ribs crunched as the retractor jaws clicked their way open. Inside her chest cavity the glistening gray surface of her lung bounced in and out.

The surgeon reached inside her and delivered her heart. In one sure thrust he punctured the pericardial sac. He scooped out gelatinous handfuls of clot. Soon the bowl of her chest filled with blood already thin and diluted from the fluids that were running into her veins. "We're going upstairs," he shouted over his shoulder to the waiting operating room crew, and then handed me her writhing heart. "Squeeze," he muttered.

The bright lights of the operating room failed to show the source of her bleeding. We toiled over her as the anesthesiologist littered the floor with empty bags of blood. I sucked the fluid from her chest cavity as quickly as he could infuse it into her veins, and nothing we did stemmed the flow. Finally the surgeon located a gushing, jagged stump too short to clamp – a major pulmonary artery had been torn away at its base. But by that time her heart had been fibrillating for far too long to be able to recover. Her fingertips and lips had become waxy and white. "She can not survive this injury," the surgeon sighed. "It's time to stop." The anesthesiologist nodded, and I reluctantly gave up my post at her heart. It jerked futilely for a moment and then seemed to gasp and stop. By that point even her myocardium looked pale.

I pulled off my gown, my shoes slipping on the soaked sponges piled at my feet. The surgeon extended his hand to me. It felt firm and solid, not at all like the bucking softness of the heart that I had gripped for the last hour. He thanked me for my help.

I walked from the operating room, my shoulders stooped, and my scrubs clinging to my damp back. In the stairwell I started to make my way down, toward the exit. I needed a break, some time to think about what I had just seen. I thought that books and movies had prepared me for the idea of a hospital emergency, but they offered images of infallible doctors and invulnerable patients. I knew about the white coat, but not about the bloody gloves, the stilling heart, and the motherless infant crying alone in the nursery. I was especially unprepared for the drunken man who had caused it all. I would likely be seeing him on rounds tomorrow, I thought, and again next week, and the next through countless readmissions. I might grow to know and resent him, while I would probably never learn the name of today's victim's infant daughter. The weight of it loomed over me, and I stumbled toward the wall. Then I put my thoughts away, shrugged my white coat on, and turned wearily upward; I still had to see about Mr. Rossignol's transfer to the detoxification unit. Introspection is not good medicine during the intern year.

26

The Impotence of Being Important – Reflections on Leadership

Ian Douglas Couper, BA, MBBCh, MFamMed

WHAT IS WRONG WITH THIS GENTLEMAN?" ASKED THE RECENTLY -arrived British doctor of the nurse-interpreter in the outpatients department of Manguzi Hospital, a community hospital in a remote district in South Africa. After a brief exchange in Zulu with the elderly male patient, the nurse replied, "He says he is important." A long pause followed as the concerned doctor tried to work out an approach to this novel problem. "How long has he been important?" seemed a good standard follow-on. "A few months now, doctor." Not sure where to go from there, he decided to get to the heart of the matter: "Why is it a problem for him to be important?" A longer discussion in Zulu followed, during which the nurse showed some signs of discomfort, before she summarized somewhat succinctly, "He cannot satisfy his wives." My colleague was musing about how one's importance might prevent one from satisfying one's wives (a fruitful exercise) when the truth dawned on him. "You mean this gentleman is IMPOTENT!"

I have often thought about this brief patient encounter on which I eavesdropped many years ago. I have come to understand that importance, or the feeling of importance, can often be a cause of impotence. Physically the phenomena may be very different, but at another level they are very close. When I believe that everything depends on me, or that I am the only person who can do the job, or that I am the best at doing something, I become impotent in my leadership and in my practice.

As I have reflected on this patient-doctor-nurse interaction, I have identified a number of ways in which self-importance can be destructive to leadership. These reflections arise from my experience as medical superintendent of Manguzi, a remote rural hospital in northern KwaZuluNatal, South Africa. The hospital served a population of approximately 100,000 people, with 280 beds, 9 permanent clinics, 3 mobile clinics, and a total staff of more than 500, including from 6 to 12 doctors depending on staffing levels. Since leaving Manguzi in 1999, I have had the chance to further reflect on my interactions while working alongside nurse-practitioners in primary care clinics in the North West province and subsequently leading an academic rural health unit within the Faculty of Health Sciences, University of the Witwatersrand, Johannesburg. My reflections are informed by my ongoing experience as a clinician, teacher, researcher, and manager.

Thus I offer the following lessons, recognizing that I am constantly relearning them myself.

1. If I feel very important, I start to do everything myself instead of delegating responsibilities. I fear passing tasks on to others because they will not do it the way I would or as well as I would (so I believe), but I become unable to do everything myself. I become an obstacle for myself and for others because I am doing too much. Delegation is an important aspect of leadership and, distinct from off-loading work, requires that I have a balanced view of myself. I sometimes believed that "my" hospital would collapse without me, yet it has continued to function well since my departure.

2. If I feel very important, I isolate myself from the teams to which I belong. This isolation deprives my colleagues of the chance to work with me to achieve a goal, and it deprives me of positive support. To gain a team's commitment to something they have not been involved in developing is much more difficult. At the hospital I worked with a number of teams: a management team, a health care team, a medical team, a community team, etc. In each sphere, I needed the support of other team members to achieve any vision that I may have had, ensuring the vision was a shared one. As doctors, especially rural doctors, we tend to be very independent-minded people who do not easily defer to our professional colleagues. Our patients and our practices often suffer because of that trait.

3. If I feel very important, I become less critical of myself and less able to evaluate myself. I no longer face and learn from my mistakes. The chances are that my mistakes will thus be repeated. An inflated opinion of ourselves makes it difficult for us to view ourselves honestly: the mirror becomes the instrument of deceit, as in the old fairy tale, always proclaiming us the fairest

of them all. I had to make the same labor ward mistake twice to come to this realization! An honest review of poor performance as part of self-reflection is the first step to personal growth.

4. If I feel very important, I am not open to learning from others. I take on knowledge, perhaps, but the most profound learning comes through the questioning that follows the identification of our own needs. It is difficult to be aware of needs if we are enamored with our own importance. Others do not feel able to reflect the truth back to us because we will not hear or we react defensively. We also do not create the avenues for feedback from patients and staff because we cannot believe we would learn anything (or are secretly afraid of what we might learn). This may be something of what is meant by the Biblical teaching, "Blessed are the poor in spirit."

5. If I feel very important, my sense of invulnerability makes me vulnerable. We know that pride comes before the fall. I perforated the uterus of a patient with an incomplete abortion soon after assuring a new doctor that, in my experience of more than a hundred of these procedures, an evacuation and curettage is extremely easy to perform. I was challenged about my leadership style by a colleague to whom I had boasted of my open and participatory leadership. If we are blind to our areas of weakness, we cannot prepare ourselves for the problems that they will cause.

Thus, I believe we become impotent in our leadership if we are too filled with our own sense of importance.

As a doctor, as a manager, as a teacher, I receive much external input persuading me that I am indeed important. To guard against this sense of self-importance, I find that I need to create time and space for personal reflection on who I am (not what I am) and to establish relationships with people who will keep me honest.

27

"Be Gentle and Be Sincere About It"

A Story about Community-Based Primary Care Research

Andrew L. Sussman, PhD, MCRP, and Marino Rivera

IT WAS LATE MARCH AND PILES OF SNOW IN THE CLINIC PARKING LOT reminded us that winter in northern New Mexico held on longer in these small mountain villages. A colleague and I had set off early in the morning to this remote Hispanic community to conduct a focus group with practice staff and community members as the first step in a study examining how patients and clinicians communicate about traditional, complementary, and alternative medicine use. Nestled in the foothills of the Sangre de Cristo Mountains, the village traces its history back to the early 1600s, when Spanish explorers first settled in these lush river valleys. As a link to the past, small family farms and ranches still provide a way of living for most residents.

A contact at the clinic recruited participants by explaining that our aim was to learn more about how local residents use and discuss traditional medicine with their primary care clinicians. This session was an opportunity to gather community input as a way to help refine interview guides to be used in the study. Based on our experience in conducting research among historically marginalized communities across New Mexico, however, we also knew that gaining the trust of these community members was an equally, if not more, important outcome.

Our contact led us to the rear of the clinic and into a small conference room. We unpacked our gear, placing the audio recorder in the center of the old wooden table, and neatly stacked the consent forms for distribution. Our participants began to arrive, and we made small talk until all six had settled in their seats. My colleague and I introduced ourselves, explained the purpose of the focus group, and asked each person to share his or her name and role in the community or clinic. Five of the six participants were female, and all had spent most of their lives in the community. With formalities out of the way, I was eager to hear from the group and hit "record."

Within about 10 minutes, I was already worried about the session. Marcos (a pseudonym), the lone male participant, had already begun to take over the discussion. Likely in his early 60s, Marcos had a commanding presence and the smooth cadence of an experienced story teller. A lifelong resident of this small northern New Mexico village, his stories were rich in historical context and depth. As the group moderator, I was initially grateful for such a thoughtful and articulate participant. Marcos, however, had already turned an introductory question about things that are important to people in the community into a history lesson on how ways of life throughout the region have changed. I was growing increasingly concerned about being able to complete the set of questions and the fading involvement of the other five participants.

I reached deeply into my bag of moderator tricks to gently redirect the conversation back to the group: "OK, let's hear from some other folks. ..." Nothing worked. After about 20 minutes of the planned hour-long session, I felt we had reached a fork in the road. I could either make a final stand at trying to equalize input from the group – and possibly risk offending Marcos and the other participants – or just loosen the reins and risk not getting answers to the questions we had come to ask. I decided to listen to my instincts and, in turn, to Marcos. He was wrapping up a long response to the role of traditional herbs in the community and said the following:

> The practice of the herbs was not an isolated practice – it was a very strong integral part of a system. Scientists have a problem understanding this, researchers have a problem understanding this, and I have to say it, and I'm going to say it this way: if you take the part away from the whole, you're taking a part away from the whole for another motive, and the motive is usually to exploit it. If you don't look at it as an integral part of a lifestyle of the people, you're gonna miss it and we're gonna end up with a beautiful glowing report that's gonna be false.

Marcos spoke these words with an unmistakable intensity, and for the first time during the session I sensed that his comments were directed at me. Stealing a quick glance at the other participants, I noticed they too were hanging on every word. As I digested the meaning of this statement, the decision to let go became clear. I sat back, loosened my grip on the interview guide, and encouraged him to tell us more.

Perhaps sensing that the group was now in his hands, an animated Marcos launched into a story about his parents, now deceased, and their roles in the community. He had been clearing out some of their old belongings a few weeks before the focus group and came across an herb he identified as yerba mansa. Yerba mansa (*Anemopsis californica*), a native herb to the Southwestern United States, has been used medicinally to treat inflammation of the mucous membranes and can be taken orally as a tea or dried in capsule form.[1] Another participant asked him to say more about it, and he responded: "The translation means to be 'gentle and kind.' So, it's the herb that you take to calm you, because it's for the heart. You have to be kind and gentle because it's for the heart. Even the name tells you that."

As my role shifted away from moderating the group, the other participants actually became more involved. The atmosphere felt more relaxed and insider jokes and nods of acknowledgment marked the remainder of the conversation. With Marcos clearly at the helm, the focus group had become more of a social gathering, and previously silent participants began to share their stories and even teased Marcos about "getting off his soapbox." As the end of the session grew near, I thanked everyone for sharing their stories and asked if there were any other comments before wrapping up. Not surprisingly, Marcos, who was sitting next to me, leaned in to get the last word. As he began talking, I noticed that he reached a hand in to his shirt pocket and pulled out what appeared to be a dried root, caked with dirt. Extending his hand, he identified the object as yerba mansa, and motioned for me to take the offering. As he dropped it in my hand, he concluded the session by saying, "So remember the name of that herb, OK? It means to be tame and tameness comes in the form of gentleness and kindness. Be gentle and kind, but most of all, be sincere about it."

An increasingly important part of practice-based research is the recognition that our efforts to improve health must include the voices of community stakeholders. This involvement has both practical and ethical implications. In terms of the former, conducting formative work with community members can help us better understand how to design our studies in ways that fit better with local needs. The latter relates to the shared experience, especially among historically underrepresented groups, that research has been more exploitive than beneficial. As I reflected on these events, it became clear to me that I had come perilously close to misinterpreting the real focus of the focus group: me. The session was ultimately an opportunity for community residents to evaluate my intentions and, in the process, protect themselves against an outside researcher potentially seeking to learn about traditional medicine for uncertain ends.

As a medical anthropologist with RIOS Net, a practice-based research network in New Mexico serving primarily Hispanic and Native American populations, I understand that our efforts to conduct research with these groups come with baggage. Every contact with community members is part of a process of continually building and sustaining good relationships. Given the fragile nature of these ties, it has been vitally important in our network operations to initiate and sustain dialog with members of these groups. This close collaboration enables them to help shape the direction of our research priorities while adding historical and cultural context that would be otherwise missing.

We are fortunate to have dedicated community members involved in making sure our research is appropriate across New Mexico's diverse settings. The local contact at the clinic who helped recruit participants for this focus group has made the long drive down to Albuquerque for years as a member of our Community Advisory Board. Using both humor and a razor sharp wit, he has relayed the struggles of his community. Through these tales, told over flat soda and soggy sandwiches at our quarterly meetings, he has told the story of a small village trying to sustain its traditions in changing times. As a result, when Marcos spoke about the lack of jobs, low wages, and losing youth to the cities, I recognized this story as one I had heard many times before. On that cold morning in March, as I worried about finishing my interview guide, my decision to defer to Marcos was based on realizing that my role was to listen and convey back to the group that I understood. I believe he waited purposefully until the end of the session to give me the yerba mansa, deciding to offer it only after I gained his trust.

In the weeks after this focus group session, we returned to the clinic to interview patients and clinicians. The piles of snow in the parking had melted and wildflowers were shooting up in fields across from the clinic. Upon my arrival, the nurse manager greeted me by name, offered me some coffee, and helped me get settled. Once I was ready, she escorted me to the waiting area and introduced me to each patient, explaining the purpose of our study. Through the brief small talk, I was now able to see that the nurse manager was telling each patient (her neighbors) another story that made all the difference – that I was OK. In turn, every patient approached agreed to participate and, more importantly, generously shared their stories about health and healing with me.

The challenge for primary care clinicians and researchers seeking to connect and work more closely with the communities we serve is to create opportunities for engagement so that we can recognize the stories that affect our work. Our research efforts have clearly benefited from this collaboration, and I am fortunate to have a personal reminder nearby at all times. Amidst the piles on my desk, I keep the piece of yerba mansa that Marcos gave me. Often, as I'm preparing to head out, I glance over at the shriveled herb and am reminded of his words that provide perhaps the simplest and most important guidance to conducting both clinic- and community-based research: be gentle and be sincere about it.

Reference

1. Moore M. *Medicinal Plants of the Desert and Canyon West*. Santa Fe, NM: Museum of New Mexico Press; 1989.

28

The Dark Bridal Canopy

Jeffrey Borkan, MD, PhD

SHE WAS BEAUTIFUL IN THE ILLUMINATED GLOW OF THE FLOODLIGHTS, as she had been a few days before under her bridal canopy, with streaming blondish brown hair, high cheekbones, skillfully applied makeup around finely sculpted features, and the fine curvature that would turn any eye. A Druse woman in her early 20s, she was a member of a secret religious sect that had broken from Islam 500 years earlier and, after persistent persecution, had sought refuge in the hilly sections of the Galilee. The large diamond ring that adorned her hand bespoke of her new status as wife, likely to the son of a leading family in her village.

Only now she was not breathing.

I sat crouched near her head on the empty road, the resuscitator bag slowly expanding and emptying in my hands, matching the rising and falling of her chest. The silent desert night moon rose overhead in the cloudless sky, sketching the outlines of mountains on either side of the Aravah Valley. I huddled wordlessly, working intently to revive the woman, as her new husband quietly whimpered some meters away. I had been called from my isolated kibbutz a few kilometers down the road as I was putting the kids to sleep. I raced, if one can do that in a Subaru Justy, up the road upon hearing the news of a reported severe accident. It had been pitch black, save for the lights of my car and the endless canopy of stars on this warm fall night. When I arrived, she already lay on her back on the asphalt, having been pulled from the wreckage. Soon thereafter, one of my nurses arrived on the scene, along with the ambulance and its driver. We were joined some minutes later by an army doctor, an anesthesiologist in civilian life, who had been on his way to reserve duty at a nearby desert army base. Driving late at night from the north after his shift, he had come across the accident and stopped to help.

The couple had been returning from their honeymoon in Eilat, the Miami Beach of Israel, the place of luxurious abandon and celebration. Their first kisses and touches still fresh, they had sped back toward their village and their new home among the rocks and scraggy trees of the Galilean hills. The car had not quite made it around this one curve, had probably caught on the soft sand shoulder and flipped. Had they been talking about their future, their love, their new discovery of each other?

ABC – airway OK, breathing absent, pulse thready, but present, her blood pressure was barely palpable, her body warm. We began CPR, cut away her constricting clothing, and placed line after line, trying to resuscitate with IV fluids the spaces where her blood should have been flowing. The regional civil administrator, who quarreled with me at every chance, save at such critical times, brought in the newly acquired mobile floodlights and illuminated our surreal scene. We worked in the middle of the road, the blacktop still warm from the departed desert sun. Our efforts raged on and on – fluids, drugs, intubation, compressions; nothing changed for the better. The thready pulse disappeared. **Think! ABCDE or Scoop and Run, Scoop and Run!!** But to where? We were more than an hour from the nearest hospital by ambulance, and calling a helicopter would take even longer.

The husband asked the ambulance driver, who was bandaging his small head wound with long rolls of white gauze, whether his wife was OK. He had been united with her days earlier after all his male relatives had taken him joyfully through the village, accompanied by drums, singing, and dancing to the wedding canopy, while the women and girls of the village had prepared his betrothed meticulously and lovingly for the moment of her vows: "I am my beloved and my beloved is mine." Now from the side of the road the husband looked toward us; we avoided his eyes.

The army doctor and I conferred; I hoped he knew what to do now. We tried a few more resuscitative maneuvers and waited. No response. We stopped talking, continuing CPR against hope, against the wisdom of the books and our teachers.

Time spread out and slowed to a trickle. The road was quiet save for the deep whirring sound of the floodlights' generator and the peaceful whoosh of the resuscitator. How beautiful is the desert wind and vista at night: all around us the parched desert browns, grey, and black of the valley, mountains, and sky, save for the inestimable stars, her pale skin, and open green eyes. The army doctor raised his gaze from the woman and said, "All is done." I looked at his somber expression and nodded without comment or outward show of emotion. We stopped, covered her body with a blanket, not thinking to close her eyes. I went to the side of the road as she was placed on the stretcher and into the ambulance. I am unsure whether I spoke to the husband, unsure of whether I filled out the accident report or let it go, or even what I had felt. Had I risen without sentiment, detached, or had I cried over the loss of life, promise, and my failed efforts?

The husband likely returned to his village, his honeymoon turned into a funerary march. The Druse believe in reincarnation, where another generation takes over from the last. Perhaps a child was born with the wife's soul somewhere that night. Perhaps her spirit will have a different journey in the next life, one that would not end so soon in the desert.

After some minutes, I slid into my car and drove back into the enveloping darkness toward my home. The community of 300 was dark when I returned, except for the spotlights surrounding the perimeter fence, a few communal buildings, and the cowsheds. When I reached my doorstep, I listened for chatter, but my wife and children were asleep, breathing softly and assuredly. I shed my bloodied clothing at the door and left it in a pile on the porch. Then I bathed long and hard – feebly attempting to clean off the pale of death – had a glass of wine, said a blessing on each of my children, and fell into a troubled sleep. Reflection could come later.

Epilogue: What's the Point of the Story? Narratives in Family Medicine

Emergency services log, October 12, 1999. A 22-year-old female, non–seat-belted forward passenger in a single-vehicle accident, unresponsive at scene, pronounced dead at 12:37 pm after unsuccessful resuscitation; internal bleeding, cardiopulmonary collapse, and possible head injuries.

The story, "The Dark Bridal Canopy," could have been written in the usual terse medical vernacular. The text of the emergency log, however, cannot begin to capture the emotions, the sights, or the sounds of that night: the woman's beauty and the quiet magnificence of the desert scene contrasted with the death on the roadway, the lost promise of the couple's life together, and our futile efforts at resuscitation – all surreally illuminated by the portable spotlights. The story above expands beyond the basic medical facts into the experience of the event, creating an opportunity for reflection, mindful practice,[1] and self-healing. For me, this story is highly personal and stands out from among the myriad of narratives that have been accumulated during the course of two decades of family medicine. Several factors are responsible, perhaps foremost being the narrative's ability to exemplify elements of the complex role of a solo family physician in a remote area: the actor and witness to the struggles of life, woven into the framework of pristine natural splendor, communal cohesion, cultural diversity, and my own developing professional and family identity.

Narratives have a central and time-honored place in family medicine,[2,3] yet it is easy to shunt them aside in the face of the pressures posed by rapid-paced, technologically-focused, contemporary health care. The need to consider the story has multiple benefits, however, and may even be considered a medical necessity. As Charon has noted,[4] "The effective practice of medicine requires narrative competence, that is, the ability to acknowledge, absorb, interpret, and act on the stories and plight of others." Physicians, when they do tell stories, have often been willing to describe the patient's illness experience, while being more reticent to delve into their own roles and deliberations.[5] Stories, such as the one presented in this issue of the *Annals of Family Medicine*, have the potential to further incorporate reflection into our professional lives and to enrich our field's clinical, educational, and research endeavors.

Making sense of stories may be best approached from a meaning-centered framework. Medical narratives can be categorized or classified in numerous manners, though certain taxonomic elements, such as narrative situation,[4] narrative structure,[5] and visit type,[6] possibly have the most resonance with our field. The four central narrative situations in medicine, according to Charon,[4] are physician and patient, physician and self, physician and colleagues, and physician and society. These basically expound on the context and frame on which and through which the story takes place. Frank[7] believes that there are three recognizable narrative structures for the stories told by those who are "deeply" ill, or by extension, by those who care for them. These structures provide the skeleton on which stories of illness can be fleshed out and include:

> Restitution stories – the preferred narrative type in North America, in which a person becomes ill, is treated, and through this treatment, is restored to health and wellness. During this progression from disease to healing, the wrong is made right, and the physician often emerges as hero.

> Chaos stories – the diametrical opposite of the restitution story. In chaos stories, deepest illness never remits; rather it only increases in terms of disability and pain, and there is no apparent order or answers in the whirlpool of suffering.

> Quest stories – the illness becomes a condition from which something can be learned. Though healing and restitution may be impossible, illness can

be lived as a quest in which learning and transcendence are the result of the journey (either for the patient, the physician, or those around them).

Miller[6] divides family medicine encounter types into routines, ceremonies, and dramas. Routines are the everyday, limited, acute patient complaints, such as pharyngitis, that can be treated quickly and generate few overarching concerns. Ceremonies, often associated with chronic illness or well visits (e.g., prevention or pregnancy), are ritualized encounters that have choreographed patterns. Dramas are the practice stoppers, such as suicide attempts or active angina pectoris, that demand all other scheduled activities to cease.

These approaches can be applied to "The Dark Bridal Canopy." In terms of Charon's narrative situations, the story is an example of a physician-and-self narrative. Physicians are shaped on the anvil of their patients' experiences and their responses to it. Their ability to respond to and reflect on pain, suffering, illness, courage, and hope may be critical to effective diagnosis and treatment. As Novack et al. and others have concluded, the physician's most potent therapeutic tool may be the reflective self, attuned to the patient through engagement, compassion, and personal awareness.[1,4,8] Regarding Frank's taxonomy of narrative structure, "The Dark Bridal Canopy" might be best characterized as a modified chaos story: the patient's suffering, disability, and pain will never remit, and the physician is unable to treat the problems successfully. In general, Western culture, including the culture of Western medicine, fears the chaos narrative because it focuses on the multiplication of troubles brought about by illness and reminds us "how thin the ice is that we skate upon, and how cold and deep is the water we can suddenly sink into."[5] The modification in the current story is that the narrative is about the chaos, where the physician, through reflection, has found some meaning in the events. This transition nudges it toward the category of the quest story, in which not only can something be learned, but also these insights can be passed on to others.

Clearly, our patients are not the only ones who are in need of finding transcendent or transformative meaning in suffering and death. This need is also acute among the wounded healers who, like myself, are trying to make sense of our own limitations and experiences. Insights and reflection on events, as evidenced in the story related here, can help physicians come to terms with the suffering they encounter and provide meaning to their professional roles, even in the face of defeat. In regard to Miller's taxonomy, this story clearly chronicles a drama. It is the kind of event that shatters the daily flow and raises the stakes for both physician and patient. All the participants in the drama, from the couple, to the physicians, nurse, regional administrator, policeman, and ambulance driver, are actors caught in a scene in which neither the timing nor the outcome can be predicted. Dramas need not always be life-threatening, but by their nature they require the full attention, energy, and ability of the practitioner. Their impact on all parties may be longstanding, and their repercussions permanent.

After this incident, I continued my years of work as a country doctor: an actor, observer, and chronicler of first breaths, last breaths, and those in-between. I served as a participant in the routines, ceremonies, and dramas of health, sickness, and healing. Sometimes I made a difference, sometimes not; however, like most family physicians, I fulfilled a critical part of my role by just being there, serving as a human witness, a clerk of records, for individuals, families, and communities. Through recording stories such as this one, I took on an oft-undervalued role of the family physician – that of witness and holder of communal memory.[9]

For me and hopefully for the reader, this story provides an opportunity for reflection and self-awareness – key tasks for good clinical practice,[1] potentially critical to both sustaining ourselves as practitioners and maintaining the vitality of our field. There is so much more to family medicine than the raw facts of particular events or the statistics of our practices or practice patterns. Such stories may capture some of the intangible sights, sounds, and emotions of our work, allowing us to convey the experience and vibrancy of our discipline and provide meaningful insights into disease, illness, suffering, and the nature of healing. This has the potential to be effective for attracting to family medicine everyone from the general public to medical students preparing for their specialty choices and provides a medium for transmitting our wisdom to this and the next generation. Narratives may also complement empirical research, education, and practice through their integrative, expressive nature. Perhaps the ultimate goal is to learn how to incorporate the insights from narrative and narrative reflection into improving the clinical methods, as some have begun to accomplish.[10] Whether we aim to change health care or just provide a record of our acts, stories may provide a mechanism for finding meaning, sustaining ourselves, and furthering our professional roles and that of our field.

References

1. Epstein RM. Mindful practice. *JAMA*. 1999; 282: 833–39.
2. Borkan J, Reis S, Steinmetz D, Medalie JH, eds. *Patient and Doctors: Life-Changing Stories from Primary Care*. Madison, Wis: The University of Wisconsin Press; 1999.

3. Borkan J, Reis S, Medalie J. Narratives in family medicine: tales of transformation, points of breakthrough for family physicians. *Fam Sys Health*. 2001; 19: 121–34.

4. Charon R. The patient-physician relationship. Narrative medicine: a model for empathy, reflection, profession, and trust. *JAMA*. 2001; 286: 1897–1902.

5. Kleinman A. *The Illness Narratives: Suffering, Healing and the Human Condition*. Basic Books Inc; 1988.

6. Miller WL. Routine, ceremony, or drama: an exploratory field study of the primary care clinical encounter. *J Fam Pract*. 1992; 34: 289–96.

7. Frank A. Just listening: narrative and deep illness. *Fam Syst Health*. 16: 197–212; 1998.

8. Novak DH, Suchman AL, Clark W, et al. Calibrating the physician. Personal awareness and effective patient care. Working Group on Promoting Physician Personal Awareness, American Academy on Physician and Patient. *JAMA*. 1997; 278: 502–09.

9. Hurwitz B. Dead notes: a meditation and an investigation in general practice. In: Greenhalgh T, Hurwitz B, eds. *Narrative Based Medicine*. Tavistock Square, London: BMJ Books, BMA House; 1998.

10. Greenhalgh T, Collard A, Begum N. Sharing stories: complex intervention for diabetes education in minority ethnic groups who do not speak English. *BMJ*. 2005; 330: 628.

29

Making Time to Write?

Lucy M. Candib, MD

PEOPLE DO NOT, OF COURSE, MAKE TIME. TIME EXISTS, FOR PRACTICAL purposes, as a linear flow, and people are swept along in it. Like a fast-moving river, time propels us forward, but sometimes we can swim hard to stay at the edges where the flow is a bit slower. So how do busy people find a way to write as they are swept along? I mean, how do people who are practicing clinicians – doctors, nurses, therapists – people with clinical commitments and sometimes life-and-death interruptions – how do they write?

The first strategy is the one that everyone hopes for, the open space, the dreamed opportunity that happens when you clear the decks. Having finished or set aside all other projects, you barricade yourself against interruptions, and work without pause for a heavenly period. How long this period is probably distinguishes your station in life, but it could be an hour, a morning, a weekend, a month, a summer – depending on one's position. The trouble with this strategy is that it means you can never do it *until* the decks are cleared, which means that it can be impossible to get to. Procrastination is the enemy of deck clearing. On the other hand, if deck clearing actually means going away to do it, then time for writing can be harder to arrange but less likely to suffer the interruptions of telephone, beeper, office, and so on. You are, after all, away. Going away, itself, requires deck clearing, so this whole strategy can be problematic if you are trying to defeat yourself.

Deadlines are the crutch for deck clearers. Once writing must get done, it moves to the top of the pile and loses its dreamlike quality of being optional; it becomes obligation. Deck clearers are responsible people who fulfill their obligations. They write because they say they would and accomplish much through their relationships with those with and for whom they write. Deck clearers penalize themselves with guilt when they are unable to deliver on their promises, sometimes finally completing projects mostly to avoid the intolerable feeling of guilt. Deck clearing seems to be the strategy of those who see themselves, not as writers, but as doctors, nurses, therapists, or other clinicians who sometimes have to write something. Deck clearers respond to the deadlines of writing groups, classes, grants, chapters, and editors; they blossom when they incorporate writing into their identity. Timed free-writing exercises[1] liberate deck clearers and teach them that all spaces are useful.

A second strategy is what I call "wedging it in." Those who wedge it in are driven to write and do it in between everything else. They don't have any choice. They earn their living as doctors, nurses, and so on, but they live to write. Medicine is their grist but milling is their work. William Carlos Williams, who saw himself as a writer first and had filled many notebooks before ever going to dental then medical school, pulled out a typewriter in the office between patients or wrote on the backs of envelopes in the car between house calls (sometimes).[2] People wedge it in because they have to. Wedging gets writing done. Wedging provides drafts. Wedging uses the energy of the moment – the stuff that comes welling up, the adjective, phrase, allusion that must be captured. Wedgers use notebooks and carry them around all the time. I suspect poets of being wedgers at least some of the time. Others wedge prose into short intervals: 15 minutes between meetings; a half-hour between when the kids leave and they have to leave for work; an hour on the plane before the pilot's announcement to shut off electronic devices. Perri Klass describes wedging: "I stay up late when there's something due, I go off by myself on a weekend afternoon, I write on airplanes, or I just plain sit in my office when I ought to be doing something else, and steal a little time." (Perri Klass, personal communication, October 6, 2004). Wedgers are economical people who hate waste. Wedgers tend to be good schedulers; at some point they begin to use overlapping strategies to clear the decks and set aside time to work on all the bits and pieces they have piled up during wedging. Ultimately, wedgers set up regular times to write because they wither inside if they don't write.

Schedulers make up the third group. Sooner or later, most writers, after trying all sorts of strategies, become schedulers, but how they get there is variable. Some find themselves deck clearing so consistently that they turn into de facto schedulers. Exciting projects can catapult a deck clearer or a wedger into becoming a scheduler out of sheer enthusiasm. Some get tired of deadlines. They are dissatisfied with the limits of wedging. They have too much fun writing to leave it in the cracks. They (and their families) realize that their writing is so important that they come to agreements on how the time fits into their lives. (Wives help here. Flossie, William Carlos Williams' wife, took care of the children at night; wives deal with the social obligations.[3] Women do better as writers when husbands become "wives.")

Some schedulers get up early in the morning, some write after others go to bed at night, some come home from work and write for a few hours with their work spread out on the dining room table. Gayle Stephens succeeded this way because EJ, mother of their seven children, accepted this strategy.[4] On the other hand, Joan Bolker, a writing therapist, says she has never known a woman who could do it at the dining room table.[5] David Loxterkamp gets up at 4:30 am, feeds the cats, and then starts to write.[6] Richard Seltzer goes to bed at 8:30 pm, wakes up at 1 am, writes for two hours, and then goes back to bed till 6 am.[7] Schedulers also create special space – a study, an alcove, a spot, a chair. Chekhov wrote on weekends in a cabin at the end of the cherry orchard behind the house.[8] (He is famous for having said that medicine was his lawful wife, literature his mistress. When he was bored – also translated as "fed up" – with one, he would "spend the night" with the other.[9] Today's women clinician writers, struggling for balance in their lives, may not see Chekhov's metaphor of a lover as useful; they may be spread between too many loves already.)

Schedulers have arrived at a time in their lives and their relationships where the questions of "if" (that plague the deck clearers), and "when" (that constrain the wedgers) get resolved into the "how" of accomplishment. Schedulers force themselves to confront their own motivation and to face off against the demons of self-doubt and procrastination. With time, clinicians who write will use various strategies, or combinations of strategies, to build writing into their lives. I confess, I am a deck clearer who romanticizes wedgers but longs to be a built-in scheduler. Schedulers ultimately find a way to invite the insistent mistress of writing into their work and family life; their spouses accept that theirs is a ménage à trois.

For myself, I still need to clear the decks and make an open space to write, but now I set aside a time to do it. This piece is a product of my Tuesday morning scheduled writing time.

References

1. Elbow P. *Writing with Power: Techniques for Mastering the Writing Process.* New York, NY: Oxford University Press; 1981.
2. Williams WC. *The Autobiography of William Carlos Williams.* New York, NY: Random House; 1951.

3. William Carlos Williams. In: *Writers at Work: The Paris Review Interviews*. Third Series. New York, NY: The Viking Press; 1967.
4. Stephens GG. *The Intellectual Basis of Family Practice*. Tucson, Ariz: Winter Publishing; 1982.
5. Bolker J. A room of one's own is not enough. In: Bolker J, ed. *The Writer's Home Companion*. New York, NY: Henry Holt and Company; 1997: 183–99.
6. Loxterkamp D. *A Measure of My Days: The Journal of a Country Doctor*. Hanover, NH: University Press of New England; 1997.
7. Selzer R. The pen and the scalpel. *New York Times Magazine*. August 21, 1988, 30–31.
8. Callow P. *Chekhov: The Hidden Ground*. Chicago, Ill: Ivan R. Dee; 1998.
9. Schwartz RS. "Medicine Is My Lawful Wife" – Anton Chekhov, 1860–1904. *N Engl J Med*. 2004; 351: 213–14.

Section 6

The Essence of Family Medicine

According to an old saying, "no matter where you go, there you are." People grow, relationships evolve, and circumstances change; in the end, though, our essence remains the same. So it is with family medicine. Since its inception as a medical specialty in 1969, there have been dramatic changes in technology, health policies, and the administration and organization of care, yet the heart of the specialty – that desire to bring wholeness and connection to patient care – is constant.

In this section, we look at some of the essential elements of family medicine and their crucial role in the future of personal and compassionate health care.

- *Personal doctoring*: a memorial service is testimony to a community's deep appreciation of its family physician's commitment and caring. William Phillips and Larry Green resolve that innovation and change in primary care should aim to strengthen personal doctoring.
- *Caring*: many of our frustrations with twenty-first-century health care are the result of twentieth-century industrial reforms. Darius Rastegar calls for health care that is not only efficient but also effective and caring.
- *Commitment*: now that corporations have replaced physicians as owners of most US medical practices, David Loxterkamp redefines "ownership" in very human terms.
- *Teamwork*: according to George Saba and colleagues, it is time to replace the myth of the lone, self-sacrificing primary care physician, a staple of the twentieth century, with a new, team-based paradigm.

- *Presence*: a personal experience convinces Cherie Glazner that family physicians make an important contribution to hospital care and must remain part of that changing environment.

30

A Public Celebration of a Personal Doctor

William R. Phillips, MD, MPH, and Larry A. Green, MD

THE HIGH SCHOOL GYMNASIUM IN THE SMALL TOWN OF CLE ELUM HAS seen all sorts of celebrations. Dusty banners hanging from the rafters remind young and old of past victories over teams from other small towns scattered across the Cascade Mountains, the evergreen spine that divides the state of Washington.

This time, however, the generations were crowding in to share, not a victory, but a loss. The town's family doctor of 33 years, our friend John Anderson, had fallen victim to malignant melanoma at a young 63 years.

We came for personal reasons but witnessed a public process. We came to respect a friend and colleague, but were drawn into the experience of a community sharing the loss of its family doctor.

Transitions test our strengths, weaknesses, and values. For a family those times are often birth, marriage, illness, and death. Now the US system of health care faces a time of transition and transformation. This national transition will no doubt bring both ups and downs. We will need to make difficult choices and important commitments.

As the memorial service unfolded, we saw relationships, heard histories, and felt community. It was powerful testimony to the value that personal doctoring offers to patients, families, communities, and to the future. By bearing witness to this event, we call upon the clinicians and policy makers engineering health care reform to preserve the process of personal doctoring.

> People draw together as they enter the gym: wheat farmers and loggers, business owners and schoolteachers, heavy equipment operators and grandmothers.

They gather from around the state and some from across the country. The people who care are there: nurses and doctors and team members from the hospital and clinic. Many are patients; some are neighbors or local business colleagues. All consider themselves friends.

They file in past photos posted on the gym wall and fill the folding chairs set out on the basketball court. The crowd extends up high into the bleachers, with a proud preference for the home team side. The doctor's widow, a well-loved teacher in the local schools, sits peacefully in the front row with her children and their children. The lights dim, a home-grown video begins, and the scoreboard wall brightens enough to reflect onto the faces of the friends and family sitting near the front.

Scenes from life appear on the wall. Early photos show long hair; later pictures show less. We see scenes from clinic and hospital, home and garden, ski slope and hiking trail. Almost every picture includes other people. Family was foremost: wife, then children, then – with the warmest glow on John's face – grandchildren. We do not get to see all the late nights and professional frustrations, but we do see John's energy and ambition in a photo of him sitting atop his old red tractor, ready to move the earth. By the end of the show, every face has cracked a smile and every eye has shed a tear.

The service proceeds with music from a hometown duet of voice and piano and a nondenominational invocation. The host introduces the first speaker on the program, a local business leader who recalls from more than 30 years ago his telephone conversation with a young doctor still in residency across the continent. He tells us how he was open with the doctor about the dismal situation the community had long faced: unmet medical needs, a revolving door for doctors (maybe 30 faces over 20 years, none of which anyone really remembered), and a hospital with dilapidated facilities, out-of-date equipment, and no accreditation. They spoke of a new program called the National Health Service Corps (NHSC) that might offer help to such medically impoverished communities. This young doctor wanted to serve in the NHSC, and he wanted to know more about the community, its people, and their needs. The speaker reports, "I knew immediately that I was speaking with a physician willing to take on a big challenge." He then tells a tale of relationships that endured more than three decades, partnerships amongst the community, clinicians, government agencies, professional societies, and university programs.

Next, the Roman Catholic parish priest tells how he first met the doctor at 2 am, when called to the home of a dying patient. He arrived and entered the darkened sickroom to find the doctor at the bedside, stooping close to the patient. The priest was astounded when the doctor silently eased away from the bedside to create a space for the priest to step in and lead all present in prayer and consolation. He shares with us the question he asked himself that night: "What kind of doctor is this who is there at the final moment in a life and then steps aside for me?"

A local civic leader – like so many in the gathering, a friend-neighbor-patient – steps to the podium. He points to a few of the photos on the gym wall, showing the grinning doctor holding a particularly cute newborn baby. He and his wife had suffered seven years of private anguish as they tried without success to have children. His favorite photo captured the moment that anguish was relieved, when the couple's newborn adoptive son was delivered to their door, handed to them in their own home by their own doctor.

A fellow physician chronicles the transformation of health care services for the town, indeed for the entire county. Dr Anderson worked until the job was done to organize after-hours care in the mountain town 30 minutes from the next bigger town (more when the snows drifted up); to upgrade trauma care and transport in this small town on the big highway; and to improve mental health services for the community suffering more than its share of unemployment, disability, and drugs. Cle Elum got its new hospital and clinic. Many joined the town's team to get the permits, raise the funds, and build the facilities, but the speaker credits Dr Anderson with pushing the stone uphill and keeping it rolling until they made it over the top. These projects required someone with John's abundant energy, faith in the future, and compelling leadership. The audience shares a knowing laugh when the speaker adds, "Arguing with Dr Anderson was just a waste of time .... He wasn't stubborn or arrogant; he was Norwegian."

A physician partner lets us in on years of back-office conversations with Dr Anderson aimed at solving the problems of individual patients with individual needs. He also recalls coming around the corner to find John crawling on the floor in the hallway, playing with a little patient. A long-time staff member in the clinic marvels at how accurate the doctor could be with a rubber band shot at her through the reception window.

A local Protestant pastor and long-time patient reveals how worried he was when he shared with Dr Anderson his biggest fear: "I might be losing my mind." He shocks the audience with the doctor's response, "He laughed in my face." He then shares his relief when Dr Anderson explained, "You can't be losing your mind. If you were, all my other patients would have told me about it."

After the planned speakers finish, the host offers the microphone to anyone in the gathering who wants to speak. Grandstands full of grateful patients just want to be there to say thank you for "being there" when they needed the doctor. After a thoughtful pause, several people rise to tell their stories of how Dr Anderson had changed their lives.

Several people have come from across the mountains to speak of how Dr Anderson changed the trajectory of their professional careers. A young doctor thinks back to his clerkship days and thanks Dr Anderson for welcoming him into his practice and into his home. That experience was the inspiration he needed to become a rural physician. A middle-aged woman who had once worked as a medical assistant in the doctor's office credits him with urging her to return to school to become a physician assistant.

Others rise to give testimony to how the doctor's reach extended beyond this local community. A specialty colleague from the city down the highway explains how Dr Anderson offered his cesarean section skills to provide the back-up essential to recruiting the obstetrician-gynecologist that their community needed. Others – from down the road and around the nation – emphasize his influence on others.

Voices chime in from church. Airfield buddies recall John's love of flying and their yearly pilot physical exams. Travelers and gardeners and hikers share their memories of Dr John away from the office. We get to hear from some of the people who contributed favorite photos to the video.

As we listen, we recall how we knew John as a special family doctor in ways that few in the audience recognize. He was a founder of the national Rural Health Association and through it connected to countless other small towns and health care teams across the nation. His dedication to future family doctors carried him halfway across the state every week for years to personally interview and advocate for rural applicants to medical school. His belief that residencies must train family physicians capable of serving all communities called him to service on the Residency Review Committee, overseeing accreditation by the American Council on Graduate Medical Education. His curiosity about the problems people brought to him spurred him to become a founding member of the Ambulatory Sentinel Practice Network (ASPN), the first nationwide primary care practice-based research network.

A young woman aspiring to be a writer approaches the podium to share a poem and brings us back into the moment. She has it written out in longhand on a paper place mat. She knows much about the man, if not so much about medicine. (She is John Anderson's daughter-in law.) Still, she understands the essence of the family doctor: "He'd look at you and know, but still/Would stop and listen anyway." She touched the heart, as poets can, of what other speakers had tried to say: "Everyone was important and everything/Held meaning. Patiently organizing the/Details, he caught the wonder and the mystery."

Finally, the host wraps up the recollections and promises the assembly Lutheran coffee and home-baked goodies in the recreation room. Just as we begin to stand, a voice shouts out from the back of the bleachers, "No. One more!" The rugged guy in worn jeans and a Filson work shirt speaks at the top of his shaky voice: "I always did get Dr Anderson and his partner mixed up; they both had mustaches. But one of you came to my dad when he was in a coma and helped us all deal with it. So, I just want to say, 'Thank you to the Doc Andersons everywhere, who practice like this Dr Anderson did.'"

At the reception people share more stories. They are still posting photos on the wall, artifacts of special relationships with a special person. Nearly every picture captures joy. Most pictures show John holding on to someone or something: a newborn baby, an elder's hand, his own granddaughter, or a favorite tool. It is his stethoscope in the exam room, a walking stick on a forest trail, or a shovel in the family garden. Many photos show John enjoying his special places: glacier-clad peaks, fir-forested valleys, untracked slopes, or the newly tilled back forty. Dr John had become part of the landscape, and the geography of the town just changed.

The memorial service was comfortably incomplete but rich with remembrances, insights, and inspirations. It chronicled a professional life full of challenges met and promises kept, of more successes than failures, more fulfillments than regrets. It also showed us a personal life full of friendships, active enjoyment of the beauties of the natural world, and devotion to the generations of his own family. No one felt the need to exaggerate virtues or downplay the burdens of being a good doctor in a small town; the people who dwelled in this community knew John and the job he did. Visitors heard what locals knew, that it all took time and work and patience. John's recurrent route to success was engaging others in a shared vision and working with them to reach the common goal.

As we departed, we reflected upon the experience we had just shared. Like everyone there, we caught special glimpses of our friend. Most of what we heard and saw that day was about years of service, days (and some nights) of caring, and moments of tenderness. We heard something, too, about his final months of courage and faith. It was not the whole picture of the whole man, but it was the vision of him that people held in their hearts. We realized what we had witnessed: the shared experience of one community to the life and loss of its family doctor.

What we did not hear was talk about technology, systems, or efficiency. Nothing about advanced patient scheduling, disease registries, or service lines. No EHRs, RVUs, or EBM. (There were a few mentions of team huddles and leadership styles, but they were about personality, not productivity.) Instead, we heard stories that affirmed that personal doctors, living in the community and practicing among people they know, can base their medicine on evidence that is richer than randomized clinical trials.

We heard testimony which confirmed that the family doctor is a reality, even in challenging communities and in difficult times. We saw evidence that people value care and the people who provide it. We felt the force of family medicine, of personal doctoring, practiced with compassion in the context of families and community. The impact deepened when we realized that this saga was local but not unique; that similar celebrations must go on in communities across our nation.

The experience renewed our resolve that – as we work for health care reform, system change, and practice redesign – innovation must empower personal doctoring. No computer, no insurance company, no hospital system can replace the personal doctor. It is not old fashioned; we saw it in the eyes of new mothers. It is not backwater; we heard it from trusted community leaders. It is not a foreign notion suited only for welfare societies; it abides in the hearts of these Americans in this town and in others.

For some 30 years, along with John, we have been on the front lines of innovation in primary care and know the importance of problem solving, improvement, and change. We have come a long way, and we know we still have far to go. But celebrating together with those folks in that gym, with the team banners hanging overhead, reminded us of the generations, traditions, and achievements that make us proud to be family physicians. It was the voice of the young poet that told us the most about John's abiding interest in people, and it was the picture of the newborn that best conveyed his faith in the future.

When we go, we know there will be friends, patients, and stories to celebrate. We wonder: When those pictures are chosen to show us at our best, what will we be holding on to?

31

Health Care Becomes
an Industry

Darius A. Rastegar, MD

Introduction

In the past man has been first. In the future the System will be first.

—Frederick Winslow Taylor[1]

The 20th century was a period of monumental political shifts and technologic advances. One of the most important changes was in the way work was organized; it was this transformation that paved the way for the development and diffusion of new technologies that shape our everyday life. The health care industry, however, has been relatively spared from these changes and has only gradually begun to undergo the reorganization that other industries experienced in the past century. It may be instructive to look back so we can see where we are headed.

At the turn of the previous century, skilled workers typically performed many (if not all) of the steps in the process of making a product and often were able to determine the manner and pace of their work, relying on experience and handed-down knowledge. As a workshop supervisor, Frederick Winslow Taylor set out to change the way work was done and is often credited with spearheading a revolution in the organization of work.[1] His innovation, which was fairly straightforward, can be summarized in two steps: the first was breaking down a complicated job into relatively simple tasks; the second was analyzing each task and finding the one best way of performing that component.

Whereas the hard edge of Taylor's authoritarian approach has been softened by some in modern management, he has left an enduring legacy of looking at work as something that could be broken down, analyzed, and standardized to improve efficiency, quality, and productivity. These principles were applied with great success by such innovators as Henry Ford in the automotive industry and Ray Kroc in the restaurant industry. The Taylorization of industry had a number of consequences. The first consequence was the increase in productivity that has allowed us to have the standard of living that many now enjoy. The second consequence was the rise of a managerial class to organize and supervise a highly regulated workplace. The third consequence was the degradation or de-skilling of work; ironically, as technology and products became more complex, the work involved in their production became simpler and more mundane. Some have argued that these changes have caused work to become for many a numbing, monotonous experience in which workers feel little connection with the product of their labor.[2] Is health care headed in the same direction?

Dividing Work into Component Tasks

The typical physician at the beginning of the 20th century was a general prac-titioner who treated a broad spectrum of medical problems. As the century progressed, the work of physicians steadily splintered into narrower disciplines. The first specialists focused on particular organ systems or illnesses. Within these disciplines, however, there was still the opportunity for continuity of care. In contrast, the most recent specialties – emergency medicine, intensivists, and hospitalists – focus on a particular stage of care and have fulfilled Taylor's predic-tion of the primacy of the system over the individual. These physicians typically work in shifts, and their relationship with the patients they care for begins and ends with their shift.

The fragmentation of care is seen not only among physicians, but also in the utilization of nurses and other nonphysician clinicians to perform tasks that were traditionally the responsibility of physicians. One example is the development of protocol-driven telephone triage systems that provide standardized, albeit impersonal, advice to patients. Another is the use of nonphysician clinicians for urgent or same-day appointments in primary care practices.

This division of labor offers some advantages for primary care physicians:

it distributes the responsibility for patient care and allows physicians to have more predictable and flexible work hours. Furthermore, research suggests that specialist care for some conditions is associated with better outcomes.[3] In other situations, however, the care provided by specialists may be more expensive, yet no better than that provided by generalists[4]; moreover, one recent study of regional variations in care found that increased use of specialists was associated with higher costs, but not better quality of care.[5]

The increased fragmentation of care, particularly the development of process-oriented specialists such as hospitalists, has its critics. Although the stated impetus behind the development of the hospitalist specialty is increased efficiency and quality of care,[6] the benefit (if any) appears to be primarily in the domain of efficiency.[7] Some observers have decried the resultant loss of continuity and argue that such changes are primarily economically driven and may hurt the quality of a patient's care.[8] Most physicians would agree that continuity of care has some value,[9] and there is good evidence to support this contention,[10–12] but it is difficult to gauge its worth relative to the benefits of specialization. While it is fairly straightforward to look at outcomes of a discrete condition or stage of care (situations where specialists tend to perform better), it is much harder to do so for patients with a variety of acute and chronic illnesses cared for in different settings for an extended period (the domain of the generalist).

Evaluating and Standardizing Tasks

The traditional physician of Taylor's time based his decisions on handed-down wisdom and personal experience. Each physician was autonomous and largely free to practice in almost any manner that he wished; as a result, the practice patterns of physicians varied greatly,[13] and many physicians did not (and do not) use proven therapeutic strategies. In response to this variation in practice, the process of evaluating and standardizing the work of physicians has received a great deal of attention. Guidelines have been developed to establish and disseminate a standard of care.[14] Integrated care pathways (or care maps) have been advocated to facilitate the implementation of guidelines and decrease practice variation.[15] Computer-aided information systems facilitate the monitoring and analysis of physicians' practices as physicians are increasingly finding their decisions scrutinized, questioned, and limited by outside forces.[16]

Part of the standardization of physicians' work is an increased attention to physicians' time and productivity. Administrative burdens and the devaluing of physicians' time have intensified pressures on physicians and diminished their sense of control over their time.[17] As a result, physicians feel increasingly pressed for time; lack of personal time and time with patients are two major sources of discontent among physicians.[18] Granted, the perceived lack of personal time might be partly due to changes in physician expectations, but the loss of control over their time is real.

The Rise of the Managerial Class

The physician of a century ago was typically self-employed and dealt with his patients directly, without any intervening bureaucratic structure. The adoption of third party insurance introduced an intermediary in this relationship, albeit one that was relatively uninvolved in the patient-physician interaction (until recently). With the splintering and specialization of health care, as well as the perceived need for more standardized care and control of costs, has come the need for more health care managers to oversee an increasingly complex and fragmented process; as a result, our system has an ever-expanding administrative superstructure.[19]

The managerial class takes several forms. There are traditional managers who monitor productivity and quality of care. There are also those who develop guidelines and standards of care for others to follow and design systems to facilitate the adoption of these standards, analogous to engineers in other industries. Physicians today are increasingly subject to outside forces and have to deal with a variety of managerial structures, including their employers, the insurance companies, and the government.

Managerial oversight and standardization might increase the quality and efficiency of care, but it also results in loss of autonomy. Physicians are increasingly salaried employees, working in settings where they have little control over the pace and conditions of their work. Likewise, the composition of their patient panels is subject to the whims of insurance companies, health care providers, and patients' employers, as well as the vicissitudes of their contractual relationships.[20] Research in the past decade indicates that physicians, particularly primary care physicians, perceive a loss of autonomy in their profession,[21] which is a major source of dissatisfaction among all physicians.[22,23]

The Degradation of Work

The consequence of Taylorization of most concern was that skilled laborers found their jobs transformed into unskilled work controlled by others and that their work could now be performed by more easily replaceable labor. Taylor famously declared that the ideal worker was someone who just followed instructions and did not think for himself. The design of workplaces and technology to use workers with minimal training was one of Taylor's goals and remains so for many businesses today.

Medicine has traditionally been the domain of independent physicians who acquired their position and prestige through a long and arduous apprenticeship, much like the skilled craftsman of the turn of the century. Whereas physicians were once able to determine the pace and manner of their work, health care is increasingly adopting the industrial model in an effort to improve efficiency and productivity. The transformation of physicians from professionals into technicians endangers the values that medicine had traditionally espoused (although not always lived up to): community service, moral responsibility, and placing the patient's interests first.[24] In the past decade, many have expressed concern about the degradation of professionalism and have generally implicated economic pressures.[25] The fragmentation of care and the increasing focus on efficiency, however, are also threats to professionalism: physicians who are focused on providing standardized services at a particular stage of care may be more effective and efficient at that stage but will likely feel less connected with their patients and be less concerned about long-term outcomes.

Even though the spreading fragmentation of medicine is at least partly a result of its increasing complexity, one unintended consequence of this fragmentation might be that the skill and training required to provide medical care in the 21st century will diminish. We may be entering an era in which the broadly trained physician with diverse skills will fade away, much like the traditional craftsman. The generalist who manages almost all of his patients' problems might already be gone forever; one observer has argued that primary care medicine could become "a euphemism for efficient secretarial work, prompt referral to other services, and conscientious monitoring of others' therapeutic plans."[26]

The model of the future could be a multitiered system of care with physician-managers supervising other care providers. This transformation is most apparent in the increasing use of nonphysician practitioners to provide services that were traditionally the exclusive realm of physicians.[27] Some physicians will serve as superspecialist consultants, and some generalists might serve a niche-market of caring for the wealthy[28] or coordinating care for complicated and chronically ill patients. For most physicians, however, the trend appears to be downward toward a less-skilled and less-valued role in the system.

The Industrialization of Health Care

Health care appears to be headed in the same direction as other industries in that the fragmentation and standardization of physicians' work, as well as the construction of a managerial superstructure, are already well underway. These changes bring the promise of better quality and more efficient health care. Physicians, however, will continue to be pressured to sacrifice their autonomy and will increasingly feel like cogs in a machine. The nature of health care is such that the devolution of physicians' work to that of an unskilled laborer is inconceivable, but physicians will likely find their work less valued over time and will be increasingly replaced by nonphysician clinicians.

Of course, the goal of health care should be to provide patients with the best and most cost-effective care possible, not to provide physicians with fulfilling professional lives. The industrialization of health care, however, has worrisome implications for the care of individual patients and their experience with the system. Although Taylor's principles are ideal for the production of standardized automobiles, meals, or other products, the complex and unpredictable nature of health and illness does not lend itself well to Taylorism, and we all know that the care of patients can rarely be squeezed into a precast mold. Furthermore, there is the danger that essential ingredients of good health care, such as patient-physician communication and personal connection,[29] might be lost in the quest for efficiency.

Granted, for those who require certain procedures or have a single illness for which the standards of care are clear, it is likely that these changes will result in improved quality and efficiency.[30] Yet for other patients, especially those with complicated multisystem chronic illnesses that require care in a variety of settings, the primacy of the system over the individual might make them feel like a product on an assembly line. Moreover, being cared for by busy physicians with less time to devote to each patient could diminish the quality of care,[31] and the general dissatisfaction and alienation of physicians may erode quality of care further.[32] A select few patients, of course, will be able to buy out of this system and pay for the personalized craftsmanship of the traditional physician.[28]

The specter of assembly-line medicine hangs like a dark cloud over our health care industry. We should all be concerned about the prospect of a depersonalized and fragmented health care system that frustrates physicians and patients alike. Although many of these changes are inevitable and some are for the better, we need to look for measures to slow or reverse the harmful aspects of this process. Primary care needs to be valued more, and the reimbursement incentives that favor technical procedures rather than cognitive services[33] need to be eliminated. Generalists must demonstrate and publicize the value of their work through research and advocacy. Generalists also need to look into other systems of care, ones that support the primary care provider and preserve continuity of care while including the beneficial aspects of specialty services when needed.[34]

I believe that the ultimate solution lays in rethinking the role of medicine in society and a departure from the fragmented and multitiered nature of our health care system. As one observer has suggested, medicine might need to "renegotiate its contract with society" and move away from "the technical model of the physician as expert in favor of the professional acting on behalf of the community."[35] The challenge for all of us is to ensure that our health care system is effective and caring, not just efficient.

References

1. Kanigel R. The *One Best Way: Frederick Winslow Taylor and the Enigma of Efficiency*. New York, NY: Viking; 1997.
2. Garson B. *All the Livelong Day: The Meaning and Demeaning of Routine Work*. New York, NY: Penguin Books; 1994.
3. Harrold LR, Field TS, Gurwitz JH. Knowledge, patterns of care, and outcomes of care for generalists and specialists. *JGIM*. 1999; 14: 499–511.
4. Carey TS, Garrett J, Jackman A, et al. The outcomes and costs of care for acute low back pain among patients seen by primary care practitioners, chiroprators, and orthopedic surgeons. *N Engl J Med*. 1995; 333: 913–17.
5. Fisher ES, Wennberg DE, Stukel TA, Gottlieb DJ, Lucas FL, Pinder EL. The implications of regional variations in Medicare spending. Part 1: the content, quality and accessibility of care. *Ann Intern Med*. 2003; 138: 273–87.
6. Wachter RM, Goldman L. The emerging role of "Hospitalists" in the American health care system. *N Engl J Med*. 1996; 335: 514–17.
7. Wachter RM, Goldman L. The hospitalist movement 5 years later. *JAMA*. 2002; 287: 487–94.
8. Manian FA. Whither continuity of care? *N Engl J Med*. 1999; 340: 1362–63.
9. Guthrie B, Wyke S. Does continuity in general practice really matter? *BMJ*. 2000; 321: 734–35.
10. Marquis MS, Davies AR, Ware JE Jr. Patient satisfaction and change in medical care provider: a longitudinal study. *Med Care*. 1983; 21: 821–29.
11. Wasson JH, Sauvigne AE, Mogielnicki P, et al. Continuity of outpatient medical care in elderly men: a randomized trial. *JAMA*. 1984; 252: 2413–17.

12. Peterson LA, Bren TA, O'Neill AC, Cook EF, Lee TH. Does housestaff discontinuity of care increase the risk for preventable adverse events? *Ann Intern Med.* 1994; 121: 866–72.
13. James BC, Hammond ME. The challenge of variation in medical practice. *Arch Pathol Lab Med.* 2000; 124: 1001–03.
14. Woolf SH. Practice guidelines: a new reality in medicine. *JAMA.* 1990; 150: 1811–18.
15. Campbell H, Hotchkiss R, Bradshaw N, Porteous M. Integrated care pathways. *BMJ.* 1998; 316: 133–37.
16. Feinglass J, Salmon JW. Corporatization on medicine: the use of medical management information systems to increase the clinical productivity of physicians. *Int J Health Serv.* 1990; 20: 233–52.
17. Morrison I. The future of physicians' time. *Ann Intern Med.* 2000; 132: 80–84.
18. Murray A, Montgomery JE, Chang H, Rogers WH, Inui T, Safran G. Doctor discontent: a comparison of physician satisfaction in different delivery system settings, 1986 and 1997. *J Gen Intern Med.* 2001; 16: 451–59.
19. Woolhandler S, Himmelstein DU. The deteriorating administrative efficiency of the U.S. health care system. *N Engl J Med.* 1991; 324: 1253–58.
20. Cunningham PJ, Kohn L. Health plan switching: choice or circumstance? *Health Aff.* 2000; 19: 158–64.
21. Burdi MD, Baker LC. Physicians' perceptions of autonomy and satisfaction in California. *Health Aff.* 1999; 18: 134–45.
22. Freeborn DK. Satisfaction, commitment, and psychological well-being among HMO physicians. *West J Med.* 2001; 174: 13–18.
23. Lewis CE, Prout DM, Chalmers EP, Leake B. How satisfying is the practice of internal medicine? A national survey. *Ann Intern Med.* 1991; 114: 1–5.
24. Sullivan WM. Medicine under threat: professionalism and professional identity. *CMAJ.* 2000; 162: 673–75.
25. Wynia MK, Latham SR, Kao AC, Berg JW, Emanuel LL. Medical professionalism in society. *N Engl J Med.* 1999; 314: 1612–16.
26. Zuger A. Nurse practitioners in primary care [letter]. *N Engl J Med.* 1994; 330: 1539.
27. Druss BG, Marcus SC, Olfson M, Tanielian T, Picus HA. Trends in care by nonphysician clinicians in the United States. *N Engl J Med.* 2003; 348: 130–37.
28. Brennan TA. Luxury primary care – market innovation or threat to access? *N Engl J Med.* 2002; 346: 1165–68.
29. Branch WT. Is the therapeutic nature of the patient-physician relationship being undermined? *Arch Intern Med.* 2000; 160: 2257–60.
30. Halm EA, Lee C, Chassin MR. Is volume related to outcome in health care? A systematic review and methodologic critique of the literature. *Ann Intern Med.* 2002; 137: 511–20.
31. Campbell SM, Hann M, Hacker J, et al. Identifying predictors of high quality care in English general practice: observational study. *BMJ.* 2001; 323: 784–87.
32. Linn LS, Brook RH, Clark VA, Davies AR, Fink A, Kosecoff J. Physician and patient satisfaction as factors related to the organization of internal medicine group practices. *Med Care.* 1985; 23: 1171–78.
33. Ginsburg PB. Payment and the future of primary care. *Ann Intern Med.* 2003; 138: 233–34.
34. Willison DJ, Soumerai SB, McLuaghlin TJ, et al. Consultation between cardiologists and generalists in the management of acute myocardial infarction. *Arch Intern Med.* 1998; 158: 1778–83.
35. Sullivan WM. What is left of professionalism after managed care? *Hastings Cent Rep.* 1999; 29(2): 7–13.

32

The Dream of Home Ownership

David Loxterkamp, MD

"Business!" cried the ghost, wringing its hands again. "Mankind was my business."

—Charles Dickens[1]

WITH ALL THE FUSS ABOUT THE PATIENT-CENTERED MEDICAL HOME, little has been said about who will own it. Do we know? Does it matter?

We don't know, as it turns out. The most recent data set is from 2001, when the American Medical Association, the Center for Studying Health System Change, and the Census Bureau reported a range in the number of independent physicians from between 61.5% to 29.3%.[2] The authors of a recent editorial in the *New England Journal of Medicine* concluded that "the percentage of US physicians who own their own practice has been declining at an annual rate of approximately 2% for at least the past 25 years,"[2] but the rate of decay is not linear. It is more reasonable to guess that we are at the inflection point in a hyperbolic rate of change, and that parts of the country have moved well beyond it.

Anecdotally, I have seen a seismic change in practice ownership during the two decades since I moved to Maine. In the summer of 1984, no primary care physicians were employed by our local hospital. In the past five years, physicians who left or retired were all self-employed; contracted physicians took their place. The medical staff is now mostly on hospital payroll.

This trend is neither isolated nor inexplicable. Graduates of private medical schools carry a median debt of $180,000; the burden of public school graduates is only slightly smaller at $145,000.00.[3] Large corporate and hospital-owned systems are poised to invest heavily in recruitment incentives, loan forgiveness programs, higher salaries, and freedom from administrative worry. But at what cost for primary care?

Ownership changes human behavior. Research shows that homeowners are more satisfied, civic-minded, and politically active than those who rent.[4,5] Their children do better in school, have fewer behavioral problems, and are less likely to become pregnant as teenagers. The differences, though not easily explained, are real, consistent, and lasting. Ownership serves as an anchor for an otherwise fluid society; money is the tangible and symbolic measure of that investment. Ownership encourages stability, upon which the doctor-patient relationship is moored. And relationships – those great laboratories of the self – are where we might finally face our social fears instead of endlessly searching for a better fit, moves some have called the geographic cure.

It's a Wonderful Life

Americans have long dreamed of home ownership. The rate rose from 29% of households in 1900 to 68.8% today.[6] Major growth began in the 1940s, when government codified tax incentives and footed the bill of social infrastructure. It was about this time that Frank Capra directed his favorite film, *It's a Wonderful Life*, starring James Stewart (George Bailey), Donna Reed (his wife, Mary), and Lionel Barrymore as the real estate tycoon, Henry Potter. Upon release, the film was a box office flop, but it became a Christmas classic in the 1970s after copyright protection lapsed and television stations rebroadcast it each season.

It's a Wonderful Life is the story of a small-town savings and loan manager who comes to regard his worth through the lives he has touched – family, friends, and loan recipients. George Bailey inherited the dream of home ownership from his father, Peter, who once said, "It's deep in the race for a man to want his own roof, walls, and fireplace." Potter knew that there was profit and power in keeping the "discontented, lazy rabble" of Bedford Falls in rental units owned by him. As a board member of the Bailey Brothers Building and Loan Company, he demanded to know, "Are you running a business or a charity ward?" George countered with his famous defense:

Just remember this, Mr. Potter, that this rabble you're talking about [does] most of the working and paying and living and dying in this community. Well, is it too much to have them work and pay and live and die in a couple of decent rooms and a bath? Anyway, my father didn't think so. People were human beings to him, but to you ... they're cattle. Well, in my book, he died a much richer man than you'll ever be.[7]

A major study of the patient-centered medical home, The National Demonstration Project, was concluded in June of 2008. It is curious that 23 of the 36 selected practices, or 63.8%, were physician-owned, a figure strikingly similar to the national home ownership average. The perception that family doctors still own their practices, or want to, is at odds with the current trend for residency graduates to take salaried positions in hospital systems.

Rights of Ownership

What will be the consequence? The culture of group practice was studied in 2003 by Curoe, Kralewski, and Kassi.[8] They found that two factors – size and ownership – were pivotal. The authors surveyed 547 primary care clinicians from 148 Midwestern clinics and analyzed their data using contingency and complexity theory. They found that clinics owned by private or hospital-based systems had "less organizational trust, less identification with the group practice, and less collegiality among physicians." They also found that "quality emphasis increases as ownership shifts to systems and their larger organizational capacity."

In my own practice, I wonder what would be different if our business plan required the approval of a corporate board or CEO. Would we have become a Rural Health Center, which has allowed us to carry a generous caseload of Medicare/Medicaid patients? Would we prescribe Suboxone in our office in response to the epidemic of opioid abuse in rural Maine? Would we allow, let alone encourage, clinicians to work on a part-time basis or take sabbatical leave, as I did to hone my skills for treating patients infected with HIV when they began to return home with end-stage disease? Would we know or care what our patients earn and can afford? Would we still be practicing here, seeing generations of patients for more than a generation of time? Would we have thought to improve our practice enough to apply for or have been chosen for the National Demonstration Project? Is it possible that it chose so many physician-owned practices because we were the ones willing to change?

My point is this: ownership influences the choices we make. And by owner-ship, I mean more than who signs our paycheck. It is a reflection of our values and integrity; it reveals who we are and what matters in our lives. A dozen years ago I wrote about the many voices that clamor for the doctor's attention.[9] We are obliged to listen to licensing boards, credentialing committees, peer-review organizations, and insurance carriers. We respond to the legacy of general prac-titioners who laid the moral foundation for family medicine, the humanists who reformed it, and consultants who now sell it with direct-to-consumer marketing. Add the bankers who hold our student loans, and, equally, the graduates who understandably rush to jobs that offer the best return on their career investment. The new hospital bosses have their own bills to pay, including for large surgical suites, cardiac catheterization laboratories, dialysis units, and imaging depart-ments. Some of us, too, are haunted by whispers of self-doubt, the call of duty, or the siren song of pride. But this chorus carries a partial tune. The missing voice, the most insistent and challenging one, the person who will deliver us to our finest hour, who will talk us through every moral conundrum, is the patient who we thought needed us.

Vox Clamantis In Deserto

In the 1960s, family practice took advantage of, but certainly did not create, the social forces that shaped our emerging specialty. So today, we cannot expect it to counter the sea change in American culture. It is certainly possible that fam-ily medicine will go the way of the family market and family farm. Even then, we can take ownership in our practices. We can be the owners and leaders of an American-styled primary care delivery system. Hospital managers will always attend to the bottom line and move to maximize their profits. Profit lies in tech-nology, procedures, tests, and drugs. There is no real incentive to foster the kind of lifestyle changes, preventative strategies, and strong relationships that makes crisis care a matter of last resort.

I also doubt that the current fashion of boutique, subscription, or Ideal Micro Practices that accept (only) direct payment from their clientele will secure the goal of a more responsible and responsive health care system. Too many patients lack the money, intelligence, and maturity to take care of themselves. And although the structural arrangement of receiving payment directly from the patient helps to reinforce the locus of responsibility, it is not necessary or suf-ficient to sustain ongoing relationships.

Those of us who sit each day with the dying, bereft, lonely, and disillusioned, those who suffer chronic pain or struggle to buy their medications, know clearly what George Bailey learned from his fateful jump: "Strange, isn't it? Each man's life touches so many other lives, and when he isn't around he leaves an awful hole, doesn't he?" I hope we will not let primary care become an awful hole. Will we be the voice that speaks for the lives we touch and that touch us in return?

Together we can advocate for reimbursement and loan forgiveness programs, admissions policies, and training sites that favor primary care. Together we must demand a broader, more-farsighted, and compassionate view of the business of medicine. I am reminded here of another Christmas classic, and words uttered equally to the point:

> "Business!" cried the ghost, wringing its hands again. "Mankind was my business. The common welfare was my business; charity, mercy, forbearance, and benevolence, were, all, my business. The dealings of my trade were but a drop of water in the comprehensive ocean of my business."[1]

As we indenture our labor, mortgage our homes, lease our cars, and live on borrowed time, let's at least own our conscience and the decisions about whom we serve. And work to create systems and structures that dignify and promote human relationships – the very foundation of primary care. We cannot afford to relinquish the dream. Ownership, by which I also mean a sense of commitment and empowerment, begins at home, in the medical home, at the heart of medicine.

References

1. Dickens, C. *A Christmas Carol*. Boston, MA: The Atlantic Monthly Press; 1920. p. 33.
2. Isaacs SL, Jellinek PS, Ray WL. The independent physician – going, going. … *N Engl J Med*. 2009; 360(7): 655–57.
3. Baldauf S. Medicine: seeing the big picture. *US News & World Report*. 30 March 2007.
4. Kerch S. The happy homeowner. It's academic: home ownership breeds satisfaction. *CBS.MarketWatch.com*. 26 June 2003. www.marketwatch.com/news/story/social-benefits-homeownership/story.aspx?guid=[2F344F23-BDE9-4CA9-91D2-2A8DF6051194].
5. Rossi P, Weber E. The Social Benefits of Homeownership: Empirical Evidence from National Surveys. *Housing Policy Debate*. Vol 7, Iss 1. Fannie Mae Foundation; 1996.
6. Yglesias, M. Why home ownership? *TheAtlantic.com*. 2 Sep 2007. Available at www.theatlantic.com/politics/archive/2007/09/why-homeownership/46080/ (accessed July 30, 2012).
7. Dirks T. *It's a Wonderful Life* [review]. Available at www.filmsite.org/itsa.html (accessed July 30, 2012).
8. Curoe A, Kralewski J, Kaissi A. Assessing the cultures of medical group practice. *J Am Board Fam Pract*. 2003; 16(5): 394–98.

9. Loxterkamp D. Hearing voices: how should doctors respond to their calling? *New Engl J Med.* 1996; 335(26): 1991–93.

33

The Myth of the Lone Physician

Toward a Collaborative Alternative

George W. Saba, PhD, Teresa J. Villela, MD, Ellen Chen, MD, Hali Hammer, MD, and Thomas Bodenheimer, MD, MPH

Introduction

The traditional image of the primary care doctor is that of the lone physician, black bag in hand, braving the elements to deliver a baby, tending to a feverish child, or attending the bedside vigil of a family's dying loved one. Whether driving on a rainy, rural road in the middle of the night or treating a waiting room full of patients in a Marcus Welby-like office, this lone physician has acquired mythic proportions in American society.

Grounded in Greek mythology, the iconic lone physician embodies the noble ideals of superior knowledge, self-sacrifice, compassion, accessibility, ethical judgment, and equal treatment for all. This myth has persisted because it represents values and beliefs that have benefited both physicians and patients and is reinforced by our biomedical paradigm, social expectations of healing, health care funding, and legal culpability for malpractice.

For individuals who choose medicine as a career, the myth promises physicians a sense of control: over one's practice, over one's schedule, and over one's patient care decisions. The lone physician maintains individual responsibility and accountability, fostering pride in work that can span from making split-second, life-saving decisions to applying clinical acumen in discovering the accurate diagnosis for a complex patient. The subsequent praise and gratitude from patients and families nourish the physician, and reinforce the notion of individual heroism. This sense of control, illusory as it may be, often overshadows our awareness of the myth's dark side. In this essay, we review how this myth clashes with the current reality of primary care practice, and suggest an alternative that places the physician within the context of a highly functioning health care team.

The Reality of Primary Care

Day-to-day life for primary care physicians steers far from the idyllic image. The lone primary care physician would take an estimated 21.7 hours per day to provide all recommended acute, chronic, and preventive care for a standard panel of patients.[1] In a recent survey of general internists and family physicians, 78% reported little control over their work, 27% experienced serious job dissatisfaction, and 30% planned to leave their practice within 2 years.[2] For primary care physicians who embrace the biopsychosocial model,[3] the myth fundamentally fails them as they strive to be super-doc – one person to attend to the biomedical, individual, and interpersonal needs of patients and families in 15-minute increments. The "tyranny of the urgent"[4] creates a work life in which autonomy gives way to isolation, continuity to fragmentation, and compassion to burnout.

The reality of primary care work life and the perception that it is too demanding and stressful have discouraged student and resident interest in primary care careers. Only 10% of US medical graduates in 2011 chose adult primary care residencies, and the number of family medicine residency positions filled by US medical school graduates hovers at 50%.[5]

The lone physician myth has serious consequences for patients too: 73% of US adults report difficulty accessing primary care services; 28% of Medicare patients without a primary care physician have difficulty finding one[6]; and a growing number of patients express dissatisfaction because "my doctor doesn't know who I am."[7] The reality of primary care for most Americans falls short of the mythical doctor-patient relationship.

Current changes in health care add to the urgency of finding an alternative to this mythology. The reduction of duty hours for residents and the hegemony of the hospitalist model ensure that future generations of physicians will no longer be the lone physician caring for patients throughout their hospital stay. The patient-centered medical home and other primary care redesign models increasingly position primary care physicians in collaboration with other health professionals on a daily basis.

As we jettison many of the dysfunctional aspects of the lone physician myth, we need to craft a new narrative of a physician who thrives within a network of relationships. Doing so will require a shift in the paradigm of how we practice primary care from "I" (the lone physician) to "we" (the physician within a highly functioning health care team). A different mythology is needed to guide physicians and society about their roles and expectations within this new paradigm.

Cultural Transformation to the Highly Functioning Health Care Team

What does it mean to move from the lone physician to a team-based paradigm? Minimally, it means moving away from physician-centered practices to practices composed of physician-led teams. Descriptions of these care teams have included several key elements: definition of shared goals, creation of effective clinical and administrative systems, delineation of tasks, development of new team-focused training, and improvement of structures and processes of communication.[8] The task for the physician is to move from thinking about my patients to our patients.

A more fundamental challenge of the new paradigm, however, is that it brings together two existing networks for the purpose of providing optimal clinical care – the patient network and the care team network. The patient network includes family, friends, and community supports. The care team network is the team of clinicians (physicians, nurse practitioners, and physician assistants), nurses, nonlicensed allied health workers, social workers, nutritionists, behavioral health professionals, pharmacists, and other health personnel. These two networks come together to form a larger system – the highly functioning health care team (HFHCT). Like any other newly formed human system, an HFHCT will need to answer fundamental questions about its functioning.

- What will be the roles and responsibilities of each team member?
- What systems and skills are needed to ensure effective communication?
- How will decisions be shared?
- How will conflict be resolved?
- How will the team foster trust and respect?
- How will the team promote the development of meaningful healing relationships?
- How will the team evolve over time?

The specific answers to these questions define the roles and tasks of each team member, and the collaborative process of working through these challenges strengthens team relationships. These answers will redefine the traditional hierarchic roles among physician, staff, and patients.

In an HFHCT, each member can take the lead on different issues at different times based on their areas of expertise and interest. Rather than physicians delegating tasks, nonphysician team members can be empowered to take responsibility for entire areas of care.

Medical assistants or nurses can assume responsibility for panel management, for example, and independently order mammograms, colorectal screening studies, and diabetes-associated monitoring studies. Nurses can use guidelines to manage uncomplicated acute infections; because most of these infections are diagnosed though bacteriologic studies, the team can develop evidence-based standing orders. Pharmacists can independently manage uncomplicated diabetes, hypertension, and hyperlipidemia; studies have shown pharmacists can do so as well as, or better than, physicians.[9] Studies have also reassured us that processes and outcomes of care can be improved by having nonphysician team members provide important components of care.[10-13]

In these examples, preventive, chronic, and acute care can be conducted day to day with limited physician input. True responsibility is being shared. Physicians who trust the team to share this work can comfortably focus on more-complex patients who need more of their time and subsequently feel less overwhelmed during and between patient visits.

Challenges for the Physician in the HFHCT

How will the physician role change within the HFHCT? What cultural changes will be required for physicians to function effectively within a team?

In the lone physician model, physicians have complete control of decisions and the responsibility to carry them out. As part of an HFHCT, they must share control and decision making. Because responsibility and accountability is dispersed among team members, physicians may fear that "if I don't do it, it won't get done," or that "no one will care as much about this patient and go the extra mile." Physicians must participate in the development of mechanisms to prevent patient care fragmentation and to ensure prompt follow-up of important clinical data. Although workflow mapping and electronic health records will form part of these systems, it is essential that we implement processes that promote candid communication and strengthen a trusting working relationship among team members.

Physicians may fear losing the sense of personal pride for single-handedly achieving life-changing outcomes for patients. This pride buoys many physicians through stressful days and nights in practice: "I saved his life"; "I feel good about how I handled that problem." Will we find it as personally rewarding when a panel manager facilitates the early diagnosis of colon cancer and saves a patient's life?

Similarly, physicians may risk losing the primary relationship with their patients and families. How will it feel to have the patient in the above example bypass the physician to hug the panel manager who saved her life through routine cancer screening? Primary care physicians highly value the special relationship forged in working with a patient over time. That intense one-on-one relationship will need to be replaced with a meaningful sense of connectedness within the team.

Physicians must be cautious not to view other team members' participation as a means to unload undesirable tasks. The distribution of tasks should be guided by what is best for patient care, and team members should be included in making the decisions governing how they will function and in what roles. Anecdotes abound of medical assistants, nurses, and pharmacists who feel a renewed sense of purpose when they are given the responsibility to share in the care of a panel of patients. Yet if the change is not done well, or if they feel that the change is forced upon them, the entire endeavor may be undermined.

For patients and families, the transformation may represent the most profound change. For decades patients have viewed the lone physician as their ticket to good health. Will patients accept and value care from other team members? Anecdotes suggest that, if team members are introduced by the physician and are viewed as competent and caring, patients gladly accept them. Little research has been done, however, to elucidate whether patients will accept the new team paradigm, whether they will accept their new roles as active team members, and what it might take for them to trust the new team relationships. How can patients and families become involved in shaping how the HFHCT will function? These underexplored questions for those who are at the center of care are perhaps the most exciting and important aspect of the paradigm shift from "I" to "we."

Challenges in Medical Education

Medical training fosters the idea of the lone physician, as students learn early in their education to take ownership of patients and are expected to assume complete responsibility to avoid making mistakes.[14,15] In our experience training family medicine residents, this ingrained expectation poses a challenge to embracing team-based care. Residents, despite integration of team models within their training, can feel threatened that team care will dilute their sense of individual responsibility, success, control, and relationships with patients. Some residents lament that their patients bond to other team members more than to them. When team members independently act in response to a patient need, residents appropriately ask, "Who's in charge here?" Their struggle with the loss of the rewards of the lone physician is coupled with the new responsibilities of working within a team – yet another skill for residents to learn. They may experience frustration at the effort required to master this skill, feeling it easier "to just do it myself."

A culture of self-sacrifice permeates medical training; for students, the high praise of being a team player means pitching in and staying late, not necessarily working with others to provide care. As our program has restructured inpatient clinical education to conform to new duty-hour guidelines, we have asked residents to function increasingly as collaborative inpatient team members. Even though they recognize the benefits of teamwork and of reducing their time in the hospital, residents express concerns about relinquishing ownership of their patients' care – missing the exhilaration of seeing a patient through a crisis or attending a critical family meeting. They worry that shift work subverts continuity, increases fragmentation, and creates opportunities for mistakes. They wonder whether they will lack sufficient clinical experience if they cannot care for patients throughout the course of an illness. The findings of a recent national survey of residents' perspectives on duty hours mirrors these concerns among our residents.[16]

What Will It Take to Support Change in the Physician Role?

For HFHCTs to develop and thrive, the administrative leadership of a clinical practice must envision this paradigm shift as essential to providing optimal care. Financial resources need to be devoted to hiring the necessary personnel and developing team processes. Team members need to be empowered to do their work through collaboratively developed guidelines and must have time to do it. Scope-of-work laws and regulations must be followed, though they will need to be reexamined so they can support rather than undermine team-based care. Professional training programs need to develop and support curricula on team-based care[17] that focus on a common set of skills. Further, patients will need training to gain skills in self-advocacy and self-management. Time must be allotted for team reflection to allow members an opportunity to examine their experiences, highlight critical incidents in team care, and foster care improvement.

Broader social and cultural factors also need to change. Malpractice legislation must accommodate the reality of shared responsibility and accountability for key decision-making processes. Financial reimbursement structures must support a team approach.

In our profession's efforts to create HFHCTs, we have yet to articulate a myth that takes us from the lone physician to the team-based physician. As we strive to transform primary care, we will need to develop a new cultural image and model of the physician healer that more effectively helps us deal with the realities of practice while retaining the special relationships inherent in family medicine.

The Genesis of a New Mythology

One place we might look for our new model is in the field of aviation. Physicians and pilots share characteristics of the highly trained expert who makes split-second decisions to save lives.[18] In the past the aviation crew and passengers assumed a passive role – parallel to how nonmedical staff and patients function within the lone physician myth. To improve safety, the aviation industry shifted its culture by introducing crew resource management, which trains flight personnel to develop communication skills, fosters cohesiveness among team members, and facilitates team decision making to prevent errors.[19]

This new paradigm was put to the test on January 15, 2009, when Captain C. B. "Sully" Sullenberger safely landed US Airways Flight 1549 on the Hudson River after engine failure from striking a flock of birds, and the crew helped passengers to evacuate quickly. The flight crew had intensive training in crew resource management that prepared them to function in a crisis. Although the pilot had the responsibility and expertise in emergency landing, without the training and quick actions of the crew and the heightened sense of cooperation of the passengers, evacuation would have been delayed with loss of many lives.

Referring to the landing and the rescue of Flight 1549, Sullenberger said, "We worked as a team."[20,21]

Sullenberger, himself a trainer of crew resource management for US Airways, notes that to ensure safety the culture in the aviation industry needed to change their mythology from the days of pilots as "gods and cowboys" to members of a highly-functioning team. He has recommended that the health care field make a similar cultural shift, training team members to work collaboratively and to communicate concerns up and down the hierarchy without fear.[20,21]

Health care is more complex than airplane travel, and the team members involved are more diverse than a flight crew.[18] Yet aspects of the Hudson River event may help us understand how a new mythology of primary care might emerge to guide us. In this new myth, the individual hero becomes the heroic team. It can evolve only in the context of a major paradigm shift in the practice of primary care, a fundamental change in societal expectations of patients and physicians, and an innovative way to train the next generation of healers. We should not abandon the noble ideals and treasured values of the myth of the lone physician but find a way to transform them into a collaborative alternative, as we move from "I" to "we."

References

1. Yarnall KSH, Østbye T, Krause KM, Pollak KI, Gradison M, Michener JL. Family physicians as team leaders: "time" to share the care. *Prev Chronic Dis.* 2009; 6(2): A59. Available at: www.cdc.gov/pcd/issues/2009/apr/08_0023.htm (accessed Dec 8, 2010).
2. Linzer M, Manwell LB, Williams ES, et al. MEMO (Minimizing Error, Maximizing Outcome) Investigators. Working conditions in primary care: physician reactions and care quality. *Ann Intern Med.* 2009; 151(1): 28–36, W6–9.
3. Engel GL. The need for a new medical model: a challenge for biomedicine. *Science.* 1977; 196(4286): 129–36.
4. Grumbach K, Bodenheimer T. A primary care home for Americans: putting the house in order. *JAMA.* 2002; 228(7): 889–93.
5. National Resident Matching Program. *Results and data: 2011 main residency match.* Washington, DC; April 2011. Available at: www.nrmp.org/data/resultsanddata2011.pdf (accessed Jun 6, 2011).
6. Bodenheimer T, Pham H. Primary care: current problems and proposed solutions. *Health Aff* (Millwood). 2010; 29(5): 799–805.
7. Safran DG. Defining the future of primary care: what can we learn from patients? *Ann Intern Med.* 2003; 138(3): 248–55.
8. Bodenheimer T. *Building Teams in Primary Care, Lessons From 15 Case Studies* [2-part report]. Oakland CA; July 2007. Available at: www.chcf.org/publications/2007/07/building-teams-in-primary-care-lessons-from-15-case-studies.
9. Chisholm-Burns M, Kim Lee J, Spivey CA, et al. US pharmacists' effect as team members on patient care. *Med Care.* 2010; 48(10): 923–33.
10. Baker AN, Parsons M, Donnelly SM, et al. Improving colon cancer screening rates in primary

care: a pilot study emphasizing the role of the medical assistant. *Qual Saf Health Care*. 2009; 18(5): 355–59.

11. Gensichen J, von Korff M, Peitz M, et al. Case management for depression by health care assistants in small primary care practices: a cluster randomized trial. *Ann Intern Med*. 2009; 151(6): 369–78.

12. Chen EH, Thom DH, Hessler DM, et al. Using the teamlet model to improve chronic care in an academic primary care practice. *J Gen Intern Med*. 2010; 25(Suppl 4): S610–14.

13. Kanter M, Martinez O, Lindsay G, Andrews K, Denver C. Proactive office encounter: a systematic approach to preventive and chronic care at every patient encounter. *Perm J*. 2010; 14(3): 38–43.

14. Institute for Healthcare Improvement. www.ihi.org/ihi (accessed Dec 8, 2010).

15. Oandasan IF. The way we do things around here. *Can Fam Phys*. 2009; 55(12): 1173–74.

16. Drolet BC, Spalluto LB, Fischer SA. Residents' perspectives on ACGME regulation of supervision and duty hours – a national survey. *N Engl J Med*. 2010; 363(23): e34.

17. Schuetz B, Mann E, Everett W. Educating health professionals collaboratively for team-based primary care. *Health Aff (Millwood)*. 2010; 29(8): 1476–80.

18. Thomas EJ. *Aviation safety methods: quickly adopted but questions remain*. Available at: www.webmm.ahrq.gov/perspective.aspx?perspectiveID=16 (accessed Dec 8, 2010).

19. Helmreich RL, Merritt AC, Wilhelm JA. The evolution of crew resource management training in commercial aviation. *Int'l J Aviation Psychol*. 1999; 9(1): 19–32.

20. Clark C. *Sullenberger urges hospitals to adopt aviation culture of safety*. Available at: www.nationalnursesunited.org/news/entry/sullenberger-urges-hospitals-to-adopt-aviation-culture-of-safety/ (accessed Jun 6, 2011).

21. Sullenberger C. *Highest Duty*. New York, NY: William Morris; 2009.

34

Dinosaurs, Hospital Ecosystems, and the Future of Family Medicine

Cherie Glazner, MD, MSPH

I SAT IN A MEETING RECENTLY DEBATING THE MEDICAL STAFF structure of a new hospital going up just down the road. The new hospital's focus would be invasive cardiology and trauma, but all recognized that patients with any diagnosis would be admitted through its shiny new doors. The discussion centered on whether there should be primary care departments in this sister facility. The general internist of the group looked over at me, the lone family doctor among the various specialists, and with a pained expression whispered that he was a dinosaur in a changed hospital ecosystem that no longer seemed to have a place for him. He wondered whether there remained a role for primary care physicians in an increasingly complex medical system dominated by hospitalists, specialists, and invasive procedures.

The internist's statement forced me to stop and ask myself whether I, too, was obsolete but either too foolish to see it or too bullheaded to admit it. Few family physicians here continued to deliver babies, and although a few more took care of newborns, very few of us continued to walk the halls of the hospital at all hours of day and night to care for adults. The question hung heavy and caused me to pause, for I loved the intensity of the hospital and being present for my patients during those sacred moments of illness, birth, and death.

As the current chief of the family medicine department in the existing hospital, I was facing a rapidly changing environment. While plans for the new specialty hospital were moving forward, a hospitalist service, comprised of newly graduated internists willing to work 12-hour shifts, had started in our hospital. More than one-half of the 100 or so family physicians on staff had turned over their hospitalized patients to these newcomers in the past year. These family physicians confessed that, although initially they felt guilty about handing their patients over to strangers, their own lives had improved so immensely that they would never consider going back to the old ways.

Resolution to my uncertainty came to me most unexpectedly. The next day my mom called; she was taking my 85-year-old grandmother, six days after receiving a stent in her left main coronary artery, to the hospital. I met them in the strange familiarity of a distant emergency department. The cardiologist, wizened and gray headed, had no explanation for her sodium of 120 mEq/L, her bigeminy, and her low blood pressure. My grandmother, who had raised four children on a subsistence dry-land farm with no water or plumbing, explained in her tired and timid voice that the problem was too much medication, but to no avail. The nephrologist would see her in the morning. She wasn't having a heart attack. Her stent was fine. Dismissed.

The next morning, feeling fatigued, defeated, and fearful of death, my grandmother confided that no one appeared to be in charge. First one cardiologist, then another, had come in without answers. The nephrologist had not yet been in, but she was restricted to 1,000 mL of fluid for the day. She wanted to know why no one had spoken to her family physician. He knew that her sodium bottomed out on hydrochlorothiazide, which the cardiologists, unaware of her history, had started six days ago. Her family doctor knew she could not tolerate a blood pressure of less than 120/70 mm Hg, but the cardiologist's opinion was otherwise. Her family physician knew her passion lay in her rose beds and perennial gardens now that water was freely abundant to her. He understood that for my grandmother to feel too weak to stand up and walk her gardens was a type of death.

With fiercely determined tearful eyes, my mother took my arm and marched me next door to the ambulatory clinics, along the same path I had walked as a small child visiting my own family physician, full of dreams of one day becoming a doctor. My mother visibly relaxed when her family doctor sat down across from her, her trust sure in this physician who has cared for her and my grandmother over many years, through many stories. He no longer sees his patients in the hospital, he explained, with the pained look on his face that I had seen so often these past few years. But he agreed to call the specialists and confer on my grandmother's case.

It was enough for my grandmother. She felt safer and death was farther away. The nephrologist agreed to advocate for fewer medications and a higher blood pressure. She returned home after two days of medication-induced illness to her brilliant roses, bright sunflowers, and crimson hollyhocks. I returned to work with my answer – the involvement of the family physician within the hospital benefits patients and specialists.

It is not the "basket of services"[1] that creates a place for me in the ever-evolving ecosystem of high-tech hospitals. It is not an electronic health record that gives my place value. Drs Green and Phillips presented a question in the Future of Family Medicine Project, "What should the family physician's role be in the future, and how can it be realized?"[2] I can answer the first part unequivocally and without hesitation: my role is to be my patient's advocate, a keeper of their stories, an audible voice in the cacophony of medicine, a translator of terms, a moderator of specialists, an advocate for disease prevention, and a master of primary care medical practice. I cannot have a voice if I am not present.

The question is not so much which services to offer to whom as much as it is how to make the work of the family physician financially and emotionally sustainable, thus supporting continued involvement in the hospital setting. I choose to see my patients in the hospital, usher new babies into this world, sit by patients on ventilators run by intensivists, and manage diabetes for those undergoing the latest technological invasion. Perhaps I am bullheaded, but I fear that the voluntary disappearance of the family physician from the community hospital adversely affects not only the health of the patient but also the health and well-being of family medicine.

I understand why many primary care physicians choose other paths. Time and money are cruel taskmasters. We desire to live fully and joyfully outside our medical practices, devoting time and attention to our loved ones. The day of the solo practitioner being all things to all people at all times might be over, but disappearing from hospital practice may be the wrong answer. I believe that family physicians' conscious withdrawal from the halls of the hospital sabotages the future of family medicine and the role of the family doctor within health care. Our absence renders us voiceless. We create the very extinction that we fear when we are missing from the bedside of our patients.

We must explore deeply and debate openly the question of how to realize our role in the broader health care system, and we must creatively find those interfaces that sustain not only the individual family doctor, but also the specialty of family medicine,[2] for the answer may be the difference between a viable future and extinction.

References

1. Martin JC, Avant RF, Bowman MA, et al. The future of family medicine: a collaborative project of the family medicine community. *Ann Fam Med*. 2004; 2(Suppl 1): S3–S32.
2. Green LA, Phillips RL, Jr. The family physician workforce: quality, not quantity. *Am Fam Physician*. 2005; 71(12): 2248, 2253.

Section 7

Medicine, Society, the World

I am a part of all that I have met.

—Alfred Tennyson[1]

Among medical fields, family medicine and primary care have a unique world-view. They not only look inward at biological phenomena and organ systems; they also look outward at the individuals and families they treat, the communities in which they practice, and the nations that shape the care they deliver. They look further, at the health of the people of the world and the planet we call home.

An awareness of our interrelationships can help us adapt to change, embrace diversity, and understand ourselves. However, this awareness is only a first step. Learning to honor and respect the places and cultures of which we are a part, while remaining true to ourselves, can be the work of a lifetime. The articles in this section explore the following threads in the web of relationships surrounding primary care.

- *Stereotypes*: the New York City subway might seem an unlikely place for reflection. For Peter Selwyn, however, a subway ride offers lessons in the limitations of stereotypes, the value of awareness, and opportunities for connection.
- *Language*: the simple word "yes" can be fraught with meaning. A visiting Ecuadoran friend and a series of Latino patients help Lucy Candib discover the need to approach "yes" with cultural sensitivity.

The Wonder and the Mystery

- *Idealism*: after three years of practice on a Native American reservation, Richard Allen lost his idealism. A difficult case forces him to face his prejudices. Over time, it also brings long-awaited validation for his efforts.
- *Cultural difference*: Ronald Pust's work in rural Kenya taught him many lessons about cultural differences in medical practice. It also left him with a haunting question: did a baby he delivered have to die?
- *Priorities*: spending billions of dollars to develop new drugs and technologies, with only modest health results, may cost more lives than it saves. Steven Woolf and Robert Johnson argue that society's priority should be on improving systems for delivering care.
- *Responsibilities*: Roger Rosenblatt, a family physician and forester, makes the case that progress in medicine and public health could be erased by rapid environmental changes. Clinicians can make a difference by applying an ecosystem health perspective to their practices.
- *Faith*: when John Frey feels a sense of despair, he remembers the trust and courage of a 9-year-old patient who believes in someplace better.

Reference

1. Tennyson AL. Ulysses. In: Stange GR, editor. *The Poetical Works of Tennyson*. Cambridge ed. Boston, MA: Houghton Mifflin Company; 1974. p. 88.

35

The Island

Peter A. Selwyn, MD, MSPH

SITTING ON THE SUBWAY ON A SUMMER EVENING, HEADING DOWNTOWN from a long day of seeing patients in the Bronx, and immersed in the careless proximity of my fellow travelers, I am struck by the random precision of this moment. A group of more than 100 people share a subway car from one stop to the next, all with our own unique histories and life paths, brought together for this instant, and then will never be together again. I also find my mind wandering over the steady stream of patients I had just seen that day in our health center, all with their own stories and life details, with whom I had shared a succession of moments, both unique and routine.

People jostle up against each other in the crowded car, pushed unavoidably by the rocking and pitching of the train, a fragrant mix of smells, sounds, and images. It feels good to be surrounded by such a vibrant, anonymous mix of strangers. I start daydreaming about the lives and stories of the people all around me. The little girl to my left, about 8 years old, I think, makes me remember my own daughters at her age, hair tightly pulled back in two pony tails with Little Mermaid hair bands, pink-striped sneakers with a cartoon character painted on them that I don't recognize. Wearing blue jeans and a shiny, brightly colored Dora the Explorer plastic backpack, the little girl pulls at her mother's shirt, fussing and whining quietly, prompting just a cursory response from her mother who is preoccupied talking on her cell phone. "I don't care what they tell me, if I have a sick day and I am going to lose it, then I'm going to use it, give me a break! That bitch, I'll show her who she is messing with, I'm not going to put up with her business, I need that job, even though the pay sucks. Ain't no one else bringing in any money right now," she snorts as an aside.

She looks tired, in her late 20's, I guess, with heavy mascara, lipstick, and dyed reddish hair, and a couple of heavy gold chains around her neck. "I'm too tired to keep doing this," she sighs to her friend, "I just want to go home and chill," then gives her daughter a small bag of potato chips, telling her that if she doesn't keep quiet and stop whining she won't get a soda when they get off the train. The little girl quiets down immediately, eating the chips solemnly, one by one. She swings her legs back and forth on the plastic subway seat, her mother absently reaching over to keep her from kicking too far out in front of her and hitting one of the standing passengers in front of us. "Why don't you come over later, bring a six-pack, I'll need it!" the mother laughs, then goes into an animated aside with her friend about another friend of theirs who had just hooked up with a guy from the neighborhood, who they both agreed was really hot. The little girl has almost finished her chips, looking up intermittently at her mother as if to make sure she is doing an adequately quiet job with the chips to still get the soda. The mother doesn't seem to notice.

I sit observing the interaction between the girl and her mother, as I might in an examination room. I make a series of quick judgments about what is lacking in this dyadic bond, about what type of role model the mother is. I think of how narcissistic and self-absorbed she must be, how the little girl may be suffering as a result, and so on. Then the mother says, still talking to her friend on the cell phone, "Well, it's about 5:30 now, by the time we get to the Island it'll be 6:30 if we don't have to wait for the next train, then they make you go through intake and processing, and then you gotta wait in the visiting area for them to come out. Probably won't get to see him till after 7, then we can stay an hour, and by the time we get home it'll probably be about 10, so why don't you come by after that? I could use a visit."

I stop to consider how what I have just heard immediately transforms the stereotypes I had so easily conjured. The little girl and her mother were going to see their father-husband at Rikers Island, the municipal jail for New York City. Rikers is a small island just off La Guardia Airport with a huge jail complex that has more than 100,000 inmate admissions per year. They are taking the subway to see daddy in jail, just as another subway ride downtown might take this young family to the Disney Store or Central Park. What has this meant for the little girl? How has it already challenged the mother's coping skills and resources? Will the father be able to get a job when he gets out, or is this the beginning of what often becomes a downward spiraling pathway that will further marginalize him, jeopardize the stability of the family, and alter the life path of the little girl? I suddenly want to shield her from the harshness of this reality. I picture her Little Mermaid hair bands against the thick gray bars and barbed wire of the prison.

I ask myself, rhetorically, why does this little girl have to be exposed to the grim mechanics of a sprawling, urban jail in the far reaches of the city? Why is this the reality that she and her mother must navigate on this languid summer evening? And then the doors open at 42nd Street, the young woman grabs the little girl's hand, and they hurry off the train. Other people get up and leave, new ones enter. The mix changes, and the train continues downtown with 100 new faces, stereotypes, and realities.

The train rumbles through the dark tunnel, lights flashing through shadows, everyone swaying together, and I suddenly feel open, aware of all the stories and history that lie just beneath the surface of perception. I also think back again over all the patients I have seen this day, about how both they and I come to our brief encounters with our own experience, baggage, and secrets. Each time I sit with a patient, it is as if everything in both of our lives has brought us to this exact moment, which can be an opportunity for the mundane or, at times, the almost sacred. Sometimes we connect only briefly, or perhaps miss each other's meaning, and continue superficially through our daily routine. But sometimes, when a certain question, phrase, or gesture opens a door, we may have a glimpse into a whole new room that is suddenly open to light and understanding. Like a glance in a crowd between strangers, sometimes everything aligns, the extraneous is stripped away, and we can look deeply into someone's soul. Random yet precise, a series of interactions, of fleeting moments that occasionally verge on timelessness. These moments can't be forced or created; the best we can do is to learn to witness, patiently, with humility, and not let ourselves or our judgments get in the way of the process – to learn to be present, attentive, and open to the story that is waiting to be told.

In my mind, I silently wish the little girl and her mother safe passage as they move through the different worlds that they must traverse. I hope, perhaps unrealistically, that they will soon be reunited at home with their father-husband who remains, for now, on the Island. But then I realize it is too early to envision such a happy ending for this work in progress; that part still needs to be written. I get up to leave the train at 14th Street and am greeted by a phalanx of people waiting on the platform, ready to take their places on the train. The wave of summer heat hits me, sweet and dense and hanging heavily in the station. The train's doors close as I make my way up the stairs against the flow of people coming down, and I watch as it picks up speed and rattles down the platform through the tunnel and beyond.

36

Sí, Doctora

Lucy M. Candib, MD

I FINISH SPEAKING AND AWAIT MY PATIENT'S RESPONSE. SHE NODS AND says, "Sí, doctora." What does this mean? Over the years of seeing Latino patients in my workable but not entirely grammatical Spanish, I have come to understand that patients will often say "yes" to me when they do not necessarily mean either that they agree with me or that they will do what I have recommended. As have many other doctors, I have come to see this "yes" response as an occupational hazard. Its meaning is opaque. If I do not get it right, I could be hopelessly mired in misperceptions for weeks, months, or longer.

"Sí, doctora" could mean "Yes, I agree with your plan and I will do what you recommend." This interpretation views these words as the hoped-for agreement on common ground.[1] Too often we take this meaning to be correct and go no further. Often, however, "Sí, doctora" means "I have heard what you are saying but I don't really want to do that; I also don't want to be rude and disagree with you openly." Left unexplored, "Sí, doctora" with this meaning leads to deep miscommunication. The patient, for whatever reason, does not feel that explicit disagreement is tolerable. Perhaps cultural style might lead a patient to hope for a more indirect way to indicate dissent without being overt. The patient may fear that open disagreement or blunt refusal might make the doctor angry or frustrated. (English-speaking patients may share the same anxieties, but on the whole they are less likely to use the deferent-sounding phrase "Yes, doctor" as frequently as Spanish-speakers.) Fear of disruption of the relationship might lead the patient to assent verbally while not truly being in agreement. This conflict-avoidant posture may derive from the multiple layers of power discrepancy (class, education, expertise, to name a few) in the doctor-patient relationship between a North American doctor and a Latino patient. However democratic I may wish to be in principle, the patient recognizes the implied and (sometimes actual) power of my position, and acquiesces: "Sí, doctora." However much I may struggle against it,[2] the power difference between doctor and patient is a reality that the patient accepts using these two simple words.

My cultural and political interpretation of "Sí, doctora" had not changed much in the last 10 years since our return from a year-long stay in Ecuador until our friend Raul came to stay in our home for two months to have an intensive experience in English immersion. Since 1995, Richard, my spouse, and I have been friends with Raul, who had originally trained as a family doctor. Now he works for the United Nations in the office of the World Food Programme in Quito; he is in charge of emergency responses to disasters in parts of Latin America and the Caribbean. Learning English would enable Raul to play a role in the World Food Programme beyond Latin America and become a more effective leader within the United Nations.

Promising never to speak Spanish, Richard and I eagerly invited Raul to stay with us during his English immersion. He had, after all, offered us unfailing hospitality as well as innumerable Spanish grammar lessons during the past 10 years. We planned a variety of introductions, classes, and social events designed to enable him to meet new people and speak English for hours every day. Of course, we, too, were involved in his English grammar instruction. When I came home from work one evening after Raul had been with us for 10 days, Richard confided to me in private that it had been a hard day. He had "lost it" with Raul.

"He keeps nodding and saying, 'Yes, yes,' and then he asks a question that shows he doesn't understand a word I am saying. I finally yelled at him and told him to stop saying 'Yes' and tell me if he didn't understand."

Richard, a lifelong teacher, obviously felt ashamed of himself for losing his temper. And losing it with his friend, whom he loves dearly, felt like a failure of generosity. Suddenly the enormous chasm of language and nonverbal behavior between cultures had opened up between two fast friends. Here again was the "Sí, doctora" problem, but this time it was not a poorly educated rural Latina from a developing country, nor was it an undocumented immigrant dependent on Free Care; it was our friend Raul, family doctor, UN official, emergency specialist, who was saying "yes" when he just didn't understand.

Breaking our promises to speak only English, we had long talks in Spanish with Raul about the meaning of "yes." I reiterated my various theories about conflict avoidance and power differentials in relationships as underlying reasons for "yes" from patients, but I came up puzzled by what it meant from Raul. He put forth the possibility that the listener, in this case, himself, nods and says "yes" when he is taking in information, but that these signals do not confer understanding or agreement and do not imply that the listener has taken in enough information to make a decision. I would add to this definition, now, after more hours of observation, that "yes" may also be a way to get the speaker to keep talking when the listener does not fully understand: "I am not certain of what you just said, and I hope if you keep talking, I will hear more familiar words and understand what you mean." (This interpretation is the opposite of the speaker's usual assumption – that "yes" implies understanding.) Here, "yes" would be typical of back channel responses, "verbal markers of continued attention uttered by the listener: examples from English include such verbal acts as 'hmm,' 'OK' and 'right.' These serve as verbal indicators of sustained attention and encouragement emitted by the person who does not hold the speaking floor."[3] Alternatively, Raul's "yes" could also be an example of what linguists call a dialogic behavior related to taking turns in the conversation.[4] Raul's "yes" punctuates the interchange, telling Richard that in lieu of taking the floor, Raul wants him to keep talking. In either case, these responses, like "uh huh" in English, may imply understanding, but clearly not necessarily so.

Back channel responses may be more common in conversational exchanges for certain cultures; for instance, Japanese doctors and patients use them far more frequently than US doctors and patients.[3] English and Spanish speakers may use them with equal frequency, but men and women use them differently depending on whether the conversation takes place between single sexes or mixed sexes.[5] Such studies do not shed light on the multiple meanings that these responses might have, but they begin to point out that power relations between the speakers may affect how such markers are used. We do not know the frequency or meaning of this linguistic response among Spanish-speaking patients of either sex, but our experience with Raul suggests that this cultural linguistic strategy has implications well beyond the walls of the doctor's office.

Raul understands a lot more English now, two weeks later, and we can talk together in English about the frustration we each feel in not making ourselves better understood. Richard and I increasingly admire Raul's dogged intensity in mastering our irrational language and grammar. And I, for one, am grateful to him for showing me the limits of my stale understanding of the meaning of "yes." While Raul's "yes" may have meant, "Yes, I am listening," the nods and yesses of apparent agreement from patients can have multiple possible meanings and require more of me. I must probe with more questions and listen hard to the answers that may indicate uncertainty or even reluctant disagreement. These days, when a patient says, "Sí, doctora," I smile inwardly and begin to ask questions all over again. "So how does this seem to you? Can you tell me how you are thinking about what we were just discussing?"

References

1. Stewart M, Brown JB, Weston WW, et al, eds. *Patient-Centered Medicine: Transforming the Clinical Method*. Oxford: Radcliffe Medical Press; 2003.
2. Candib LM. *Medicine and the Family: A Feminist Perspective*. New York, NY: Basic Books; 1995.
3. Ohtaki S, Ohtaki T, Fetters MD. Doctor-patient communication: a comparison of the USA and Japan. *Fam Pract*. 2003; 20: 276–82.
4. Hall JA. *Non-Verbal Sex Differences: Communication Accuracy and Expressive Style*. Baltimore, Md: Johns Hopkins University Press; 1984.
5. Feke MS. Effects of Native Language and Sex on Back Channel Behavior. In: Sayahi L, Ed. *Selected Proceedings from the First Workshop on Spanish Sociolinguistics*. Somerville, MA: Cascadilla Proceedings Project; 2003. pp. 96–106.

37

Stuck in the Mud

Richard E. Allen, MD, MPH

UNIT 2 IS OUT OF SERVICE, REQUESTING BACKUP."

The ambulance call came just as I arrived in our rural emergency department, and I wondered what "out of service" meant for my patient.

"Unit 2, say again," the dispatcher replied.

"Jim, I'm up to the rims in mud out here. Send out a truck or something."

Minutes earlier I was sitting at home waiting for the usual phone call. Every couple of hours I'd be called to drive in and see the lineup of non-emergency visits: runny noses, drunks, empty pill bottles. Still, each call night was stressful and unpredictable because of this occasional urgent call from a scared nurse.

"Fifteen-year-old, bleeding pretty bad, don't know how far along she is; nobody knew she was pregnant." The nurse stumbled through the presentation. "EMS has gone out but is probably 30 minutes away."

"Okay; I'll be right there," I responded, "and somebody call to see if Nelson is around just in case we need help."

Dr Nelson retired several years ago. Officially an obstetrician, he was trained in the days when you could do a little of everything, from appendectomies to setting bone fractures. Now the small town was left with family physicians for all deliveries, and it was an hour to the big city for surgical backup. But Nelson was still available if you could find him, out on his horse or down at the old theater.

The obstetric nurse met me in the ER. "I've got the fetal monitor here, ampicillin, forceps, whatever you need." Marilyn was competent and confident. "Should we plan to deliver down here, or do you want to go up to the labor room?" Delivery had never occurred to me, as I thought we were dealing with a first trimester bleed. That's when the call came in.

"Unit 2 is out of service, requesting backup …."

"You'd better go out there," Marilyn warned. "They won't manage this well."

It took a moment for her words to sink in, proposing that I go out and rescue this girl. Two feet of April snow was melting rapidly, covering everything in thick Montana mud. One ambulance was already stuck, and another with me in it could put us all in deep. But most of all, it was the reservation: hundreds of square miles of littered farms, poor roads, and wasteland. Ten thousand people lived out there, surviving on a little farm income and a lot of government handouts. Some said there were thousands of rifles cached out there, though in four years of emergency call I'd never once seen a gunshot wound. Technically our town was on their land, "between the two rivers," as the original treaty acknowledged. But in the past century the town and surrounding ranch land was somehow carved out of what was theirs.

The majority of my patients were Native American, and just a few years earlier I was excited by the opportunity to serve them as I finished residency. Here was a third world country on the outskirts of my wife's home town, offering me the opportunity to aid the underserved without living in a tent or exposing my kids to exotic infections. Just like the African charity advertisements, I pictured myself lifting children from the muddy squalor, immunizing them, feeding them, and even dancing to the drums of their ancient heritage.

But in three years my idealism waned, and my enthusiasm dried up. Hair-spray drunks vomiting blood at 3 am. An insatiable demand for codeine. Baby-bottle tooth decay. Fatherless children of teenaged mothers, adopted by obese diabetic grandmothers. Beer-bottle lacerations a foot long. I was overwhelmed, and my hope in being a savior to the third world nation turned instead to resentment of being there at all. Swamped by everyday medical problems, I could not even begin to deal with the poverty, racial tensions, and poor public health. Nor would my own prejudices allow me to "dance to the drums" and be a part of their culture.

"Hospital emergency, have you got a doctor there?" The radio again.

"Go ahead Randy; what's up?" I replied.

"Doc, your gal here's in real trouble," the police officer said. "There's a little baby foot coming out of this girl's ... um, groin area."

"Footling breech," I said to Marilyn. "Randy, hold that foot in. I'll be right there."

I rode in the front of the ambulance so I wouldn't get dizzy and so I could think. We passed through town on our way to the highway. A dead looking town, I had always told my wife when we visited. It was typical of a farm town that size, with 50-year-old decrepit buildings greeting visitors as they drove through the one stoplight. The Cahoon Hotel, a dilapidated, abandoned brick structure, was now a hotspot for drug deals. Scruffy-looking Native American men hung out there and watched the cars go by. Their seemingly untroubled daily life stood in stark contrast to my urgency and my desire to help their people. Perhaps not unlike the meeting of our cultures two centuries ago.

I recalled a paper I wrote in graduate school criticizing the Tribal Council for the alcohol problem on the reservation. Council members should abstain from drink, I asserted, and widely expand the school-based prohibition programs. My public health professor called me in to talk about the paper. "Have you ever taken a course in 'cultural competence'?" she asked. It was the first time I'd heard the term, but the implication that I was incompetent at something was insulting. She never graded the paper. I passed the class but was frustrated that my term paper received no marks – like an unsigned treaty with uncertain terms.

Darkness set in as the ambulance moved along. The reservation was a treacherous place to drive, even on good paved roads. Horses and cattle roamed freely and often wandered onto the lonely highway. Drunk drivers were common, and pickup cabs were often crammed with six or eight passengers. Snow covered the trash most of the year, but now as spring came on, you could see entire fence lines covered with Dairy Queen cups and grocery bags. I was eager to live and serve there after residency, but more recently I daydreamed of cozy monotonous clinics in the city where my friends worked.

We finally arrived at the scene, a muddy access road with a collection of police waving us down. They led me to a 4-wheel-drive truck and opened the doors. The girl was unclothed, streaked with blood and dirt, lying in fetal position with her legs tightly closed. Despite pain and fear, she remained calm and silent. For nine months she had been silent, disguising an unwanted pregnancy beneath baggy clothes and feigned illness. We loaded her carefully onto the padded gurney and into the ambulance. I crouched next to her and put my gloved hand between her legs, holding back a footling breech and hoping we'd make it to the hospital before the umbilical cord prolapsed.

Marilyn covered her with two blankets, then checked and reassured me that the fetal heart tones were normal. She put an oxygen mask on the girl and then started to massage her back and whisper in her ear. Belinda was her name, the nurse told me. I sat there bewildered, my mind racing with thoughts of what to do in case of hemorrhage. Belinda embodied all that I had come to hate about the reservation: the dearth of preventive medicine, rampant promiscuity and drug abuse, and my own inability to befriend and aid an ailing people. Here was the child that I pictured, needing a nursing father to lift and nourish her. Instead, I had become angry and distant, resenting my ineffective role in the slew of medical crises.

Dr Nelson and a dozen others helped us out of the ambulance and into the labor suite. "Poor girl," he said to me later. "No support all this time." He, too, stayed near her head and whispered comfort to her, while I held on and wished that he would assume care at her pelvis.

"It's just a simple upside-down delivery," he said when we were all set up. "Here we go now." He placed my hands on both of the infant legs, emphasizing that it was *my* procedure to perform. The body was out easily. "Now sweep for the arms," he said, as he guided me along. Next was the forceps application, a bit trickier in breech than in the few cases of cephalic presentation where I had used them. "And just an easy pull," he continued. It was effortless in his hands: out came a remarkably healthy baby boy, and with his first cry the room filled with excitement and applause. Still the teenage girl said nothing and had cried neither in joy nor in pain through the entire event.

I never saw her again. In fact, I had never really seen her. We hadn't spoken to each other at all. The usual doctor-patient bond from sharing this matchless experience was entirely absent, not only with Belinda but with all my Native American patients. There was an ethnic wall I'd never breached despite my initial good intentions. I was supposed to love the people and serve them, just like the altruistic ads that had inspired me during training. Instead, I saw my prejudices for the first time. I felt angry, frustrated, and powerless to resolve the social and medical ills pervading the rural area.

The girl's grandmother was in my office almost a year later to refill arthritis medications when her own doctor was out of town. After the moment it took me to realize who she was, suddenly the whole incident came flooding over me. She spoke only a few words in broken English, confirming that she was raising the boy as her own. I wanted her to say more. I wanted someone to validate that my work had meaningful purpose, if not to save a nation then at least to help a scattered few. Cultural competence may never be my achievement, but service can not possibly be worthless.

She started to leave, then turned back and smiled, nodding to me. "You came to us," she said. "You came."

38

Indication

Ronald E. Pust, MD

SATURDAY HOSPITAL ROUNDS ON ALL THE WARDS WERE FINALLY finished as the equatorial sun reached its noonday zenith. Rainy season had begun. Toddlers, now febrile or even comatose from malaria, filled the children's ward. In the adult wards rural folks recovering in traction from trauma or post-op from typhoid perforations were joined by their less fortunate friends, village neighbors diminished by AIDS, manifest most often as tuberculosis.

By noon I had finished rounds for all the patients. The clinical officers would cover admitting at the Casualty Department of this 80-bed Lugulu Friends' (Quaker) Hospital in rural western Kenya. As the only doctor on the station, I looked forward to a restful afternoon, punctuated only, I hoped, by the predictable late afternoon tropical downpour, a staccato snare-drummer on the zinc roof, interrupted at intervals by the kettledrum – a mango tumbling from its tree above the doctor's house.

At 12:30 pm the rain was still hours away when Mrs C, a 21-year-old farmer's wife, emerged on a makeshift stretcher through the sliding door of a *matatu* (minivan). I could find no referral note from her health center on the lower slopes of Mount Elgon near the Uganda border. But Mrs C told us this was her first pregnancy, and that she was nine months along – and more than ready to have her baby!

What Mrs C Said

Mrs C said her waters broke at 8 pm, followed by labor pains at 10 pm on Friday, the night before. Heeding the nurse-midwife's advice to first-time mothers that she heard at all four of her prenatal visits, she and her husband came promptly, arriving just before midnight at the Mt Elgon health center. Mr C told us that the midwife used her hands and ears to monitor his wife's contractions, and, after her vaginal examinations, she had put a circle and an X on a paper graph every four, and then every two hours. But at 10 am, after 12 hours of labor, the midwife had told them to go to the Lugulu Friends' Hospital.

On arrival at Lugulu, Mrs C's vital signs were all normal. She seemed tired from her lengthy labor and the jostle of the *matatu* journey, but calm in the knowledge that now she would soon become a mother. Lugulu's certified midwife, the best of all external fetal monitors, with her hand on Mrs C's uterus, reported fairly strong contractions, lasting 50 seconds about every three minutes.

The midwife and I agreed that our findings during the patient's abdominal examination were normal. The baby's head was vertex (down), and we heard its heartbeat best in the mother's right lower quadrant at 140 to 150 beats per minute with good variability. Still, as the midwife felt the next contraction, pressing her Pinard ear trumpet firmly to the lower uterine area, she heard the fetal heart rate at 90 to 96 beats per minute late in the contraction. And again with the next contraction … and the next.

By Leopold's maneuvers, used in Commonwealth and other nations to determine descent of the baby toward the birth canal, I judged only two-fifths of the head to be above the pelvic brim, and, thus, engaged in the pelvis. External examination showed thin meconium at the swollen vaginal outlet, but no bleeding.

On an internal vaginal examination, the cervix was fully dilated, the fetal head was right occiput anterior and had descended to the ischial spines, confirming engagement – all reassuring findings. During the infant's journey through this first stage of labor, however, its skull had become considerably molded, conforming to the birth canal. More ominously, there was not the least descent with the strong next contraction … or the one after that. The molding and failure to descend, coupled with Mrs C's long, exhausting labor, made it unlikely that motherhood would come without help. And the deceleration of the fetal heartbeat near the end of each contraction made rapid help imperative.

What I Said

Mrs C fulfilled all the classical criteria for symphysiotomy, a procedure in which, after local anesthesia, the clinician uses a scalpel to cut through the cartilage of the pubic symphysis while two assistants hold the mother's legs, allowing the pelvis to open 2 to 3 cm, leading to prompt delivery of the baby.[1,2] I first checked the vacuum extractor, which might have helped me to pull the baby's head through the birth canal. It leaked. Not an auspicious time to repair it – and with the skull molding, I judged vacuum extraction unlikely to be successful. Meantime the ward midwife started intravenous fluids and placed the urethral catheter, the first essential step for symphysiotomy. If the carefully defined criteria (indications) are met, symphysiotomy, which is relatively rapid and simple,[3,4] can be done in the labor ward in an emergency.[5,6] In contrast, in some facilities where cesarean section is available, it may take considerable time to assemble the operating team. This was certainly true here in Lugulu – and especially on a Saturday. To be optimally prepared to resuscitate her baby, however, we wheeled Mrs C to the nearby operating room. With the indications for symphysiotomy clearly fulfilled, I now expected that her baby would soon be born and, I hoped, despite the late decelerations, would be healthy.

She and her husband would not fear to bear her next child at the small health center near their isolated farm, secure in the knowledge she had no cesarean section scar on her uterus that might rupture if the next delivery were as prolonged and difficult as this one. Indeed, as I briefly explained to Mrs C, her next delivery might well be much easier, with the slightly, yet definitely, larger pelvis that results from symphysiotomy.[7]

On our arrival in the operating room, the lone surgical technician on duty was incredulous at my explanation of how few and simple are the instruments needed for symphysiotomy. Having carried from the labor ward a routine delivery pack, I asked now only for lidocaine, a 10-mL syringe, a number 20 scalpel, and two assistants to stabilize Mrs C's thighs in the stirrups, preventing them from coming together after the division of the symphysis.[7] Instead, with some bewilderment, the surgical technician began to open a cesarean section pack.

At this point, the on-call nurse left for the adjacent room, where there was a telephone.

What Matron Said

Within a few minutes, the hospital's head nurse – the Matron – appeared and recommended a cesarean section (C-section). When I again explained extremely briefly these classic indications for this simple procedure, Matron responded that if a mother has difficulty delivering vaginally, we are to perform a C-section – and that she had just sent out a call for the full weekend operating room team. This firm and apparently immutable policy, Matron said, emanated from the medical director of the hospital, who a few years before had completed his residency in surgery at Kenyatta National Teaching & Referral Hospital at the University of Nairobi. We worked together daily but had never discussed this scenario. He was away in his hometown for the weekend.

With little to do while the operating room team slowly assembled, I weighed Matron's measured words, the authority they calmly conveyed. Silently, I reviewed the indications. I considered Mrs C, her baby, her husband, their arduous journey, their trust. I knew that I was a welcome guest, yet still a stranger, in this land. Should I "speak in the house of my hosts?"[8]

I did not speak. We proceeded with the C-section.

The anesthetic technician, on call instead of the nurse anesthetist, chose to use inhalational general, rather than a spinal anesthesia. With the aid of a nursing assistant pushing up the head vaginally, we delivered from the lower segment incision an infant boy, who appeared to be full-term. He was blue and floppy with an Apgar score of three. I handed him to the anesthetist and his nursing assistant. All the items for neonatal resuscitation were at hand; however, neither nurse appeared to be as competent in neonatal resuscitation as the regular weekday operating room team.

I waited in vain for a cry, any sign of activity from Kenya's newest citizen on this stultifying Saturday. …

Had we done a symphysiotomy, I knew in my heart, the procedure would have delivered this child many minutes earlier.[9] I could then have turned to assist the nurse in reviving the baby.

Instead, I was at the operating table trying to control the considerable uterine bleeding. The hemorrhage abated somewhat with ergotamine and fundal massage. Still, Mrs C's blood pressure fell to 90/70 mm Hg. Her pulse rose to 150 beats per minute. Fortunately, instead of the chronic anemia of many mothers in the tropics, her admission hemoglobin had been 15.9 g/dL. Likely, this high concentration resulted from a combination of the effects of dehydration from her long labor and the mild anoxia of the 7,500-foot elevation of her village, well above malaria transmission. She was strong and healthy, without the "maternal depletion" that often develops with serial pregnancies. This full-term baby boy was Mrs C's first.

He died.

Some bleeding continued as I closed the lower segment uterine incision. By this time I estimated a blood loss of 1,500 mL, which we replaced with two units of blood and 500 mL of saline. Further fortified by oxytocin and more ergometrine, the vital signs of Mrs C, the would-be mother, now stabilized near normal. As I closed her abdominal incision, I inflicted on myself the only needle-stick injury of my year in Kenya. The patient's blood drawn at that point had a hemoglobin of 12.9 g/dL – nearly normal.

I awaited the results of her human immunodeficiency virus (HIV) test.

Mrs C vomited as her breathing tube was being removed. The anesthetist, with his full attention back on Mrs C after the failed resuscitation, successfully suctioned her airway. Now conscious enough to see her dead firstborn son, Mrs C was wheeled on a gurney back to the postpartum ward, "in stable condition." Or so I wrote.

What Boaz Said

Some weeks later, I was back at Moi University in Eldoret. Now it was near the end of my year in the fledgling Family Medicine Division at Kenya's newer medical school, on the western edge of the Great Rift Valley. I narrated this experience to the head of the Department of Reproductive Health (obstetrics & gynaecology), Dr Boaz Nyunya-Otieno. Like all Kenyan obstetricians, and indeed all Kenyan specialists, he had completed his residency training at Kenyatta National Hospital in Nairobi. Familiar with the medical literature and the indications for symphysiotomy, and certainly experienced in situations such as Mrs C's, Dr Nyunya recounted why, despite his qualifications and experience, he had never performed the procedure.

When the University of Nairobi medical school, Kenya's first, was founded in 1967, four years after independence, its founding faculty members were virtually all expatriate, mostly British. Some of the enduring advances in obstetrics had emanated from this university and others like it in Africa. Among the most well-known contributions of the British professor and head of the Department of Obstetrics-Gynaecology at Nairobi was his refinement of the technique, indications – and contraindications – for symphysiotomy.

So why, I asked, given their renowned mentor, were the graduates of his obstetrics department loathe to perform his signature procedure, even when all the well-defined indications were met?

The reason, responded Dr Nyunya, had little to do with evidence, experience, or opportunity, and everything to do with human relationships, power, and authority, particularly as Kenyan professionals emerged in those early years after independence. The professor's obstetrics residents (registrars) read the same medical literature as did he. In contrast to the professor, however, they questioned why they should be learning symphysiotomy, long abandoned in Europe – and considered by some in the developed nations as outmoded, or even barbaric.

When the professor retorted, citing his experiential evidence for the procedure's utility when presented with indications such as Mrs C's, his understudies saw him as high-handed, inflexible, and authoritarian – in short, colonial. But the prestigious authority of professors, at least in that time and place, had the virtual force of fiat, and to a degree it still does. So the rising stars among these new Kenyan obstetricians, chafing under these pronouncements, bided their time.

Not many years later, the professor and most of his expatriate faculty colleagues moved on to other British Commonwealth nations or returned home to the United Kingdom. Thus did symphysiotomy suffer its reversal of fortune in East Africa. Shortly after the departure of that professor, the senior Kenyan obstetrician, now the new professor, issued an edict. No less authoritarian than that of his resented mentor, he pronounced symphysiotomy a primitive procedure forced upon Africa by the colonialists – and unworthy of his new and advancing nation.

What Does this Story Say?

That was what Boaz told me. What did he teach me? As I now reflect, I believe this story is not about Africa; it's not about gurus – good or bad; ultimately it's not even about symphysiotomy.

It's a Story about Attitudes – Not Africa

Most who read this likely will not work in Africa, but the issues raised by this experience are not about any specific place, person, or period. Authoritarian attitudes, arrogance, and the acrimony they engender can be vertically transmissible to the next generation anywhere in the world. They can poison the waters of collegiality and enlightened enquiry.

It's a Story about Being a Guest – Not a Guru

Being a guest in another nation – or on anyone else's turf – is more challenging than being a guru, however enlightened or expert. Faced with the situation just described, what is a guest to do? Act in what we may believe to be the best interest of the patient involved, or respect the edict of our host? Do guests over time earn the right, or even incur a duty, to disagree with their hosts? If so, how long might that take to evolve? It took me six years as a general practitioner working for the community's hospital board in Papua New Guinea, before I felt I had perhaps earned a duty to disagree.[10]

It's a Story about Science – Not Symphysiotomy

If universal evidence undergirds so-called best practices, why do our clinical decisions differ, dependent, it would seem, on time, place, and person? Why does science have controversies rather than universal agreement?

The 2010 Cochrane analysis, recognizing the "controversy surrounding the use of symphysiotomy" but finding no randomized trials, calls on "professional and global bodies [to] provide guidelines."[11] Meanwhile, according to the best international meta-analyses,[12,13] the advantages of symphysiotomy are incontrovertible when specific, well-defined indications are present.

Is it merely incidental that, like much of evidence-based medicine, these reviews were assembled by physicians from developed nations? Was the new Kenyan professor of obstetrics right when he pronounced symphysiotomy a primitive procedure invented by colonialists for the colonies?

Among the most recent examples of this symphysiotomy dichotomy is the 2010 publication by the American Academy of Family Physicians of a new adaptation of the respected course and guide to emergencies in childbirth, *Advanced Life Support in Obstetrics* (ALSO), widely used by resident and practicing family doctors in North America. This adaptation of ALSO, for use in developing nations, is called *Global ALSO. Global ALSO* has a chapter on symphysiotomy.[14] The North American version does not. Although there are highly defensible reasons for both versions, a divide does persist.

Did a baby die in Kenya because I did not insist on symphysiotomy?

References

1. Seedat E, Crichton D. Symphysiotomy. Technique, indications and limitations. *Lancet*. 1962; 279: 554–59.
2. Crichton D, Clarke G. Symphysiotomy: indications and contraindications. *S Afr J Obstet Gynaecol*. 1966; 4: 76–79.
3. Gebbie DA. Symphysiotomy. *Trop Doct*. 1974; 4(2): 69–75.
4. Quinlan D. Symphysiotomy. In: Hankins G, Clark S, Cunningham F, Gilstrap L, eds. *Operative Obstetrics*. New York, NY: Appleton & Lange; 1995. pp. 89–92.
5. Pust RE, Hirschler RA, Lennox CE. Emergency symphysiotomy for the trapped head in breech delivery: indications, limitations and method. *Trop Doct*. 1992; 22(2): 71–75.
6. Wykes CB, Johnston TA, Paterson-Brown S, Johanson RB. Symphysiotomy: a lifesaving procedure. *BJOG*. 2003; 110(2): 219–21.
7. Lennox C. Difficult labour. In: Lawson J, Harrison K, Bergstrom S, eds. *Maternity Care in*

Developing Countries. London: Royal College of Obstetrics & Gynaecology Press; 2001. pp. 198–99.

8. Joinet B. I speak in the house of my hosts. *Lumen Vitae*. 1974; 29: 587–603.

9. Mola GD. Symphysiotomy or caesarean section after failed trial of assisted delivery. *P N G Med J*. 1995; 38(3): 172–77.

10. Pust R. *Community Health Perspectives in the Third World*. Papua New Guinea: The Melanesian Institute Point; 1982. 1 pp. 162–80.

11. Hofmeyr GJ, Shweni PM. Symphysiotomy for feto-pelvic disproportion. *Cochrane Database Syst Rev*. 2010; 10(Issue 10): CD005299.

12. Björklund K. Minimally invasive surgery for obstructed labour: a review of symphysiotomy during the twentieth century (including 5000 cases). *BJOG*. 2002; 109(3): 236–48.

13. Verkuyl DA. Think globally act locally: the case for symphysiotomy. *PLoS Med*. 2007; 4(3): e71.

14. Pust R. Symphysiotomy. In: *Global ALSO*. American Academy of Family Physicians, 2010. www.aafp.org/also.

39

The Break-Even Point

When Medical Advances are Less Important than Improving the Fidelity with Which They Are Delivered

Steven H. Woolf, MD, MPH, and Robert E. Johnson, PhD

Introduction

Although modern medicine can be proud of its successes in the prevention and treatment of disease, much more can be done to alleviate morbidity and premature mortality. Two transcendent problems predominate. First, available care is not delivered well: Americans do not always obtain the interventions that would improve their health or prevent illness. By one account, Americans receive only 55% of recommended health care services.[1] Gaps in delivery are even greater for the poor and for racial and ethnic minorities.[2] Second, the interventions that Americans do receive have limited efficacy in improving outcomes. More lives could be saved by developing better drugs, technologies, and procedures. In effect, society faces a choice between these two strategies for bettering health and must strike a prudent balance in how many resources it allocates to each endeavor.

Fidelity

The first endeavor addresses what might be described as the *fidelity* of health care. Independent of the efficacy or effectiveness of interventions, fidelity is the extent to which the system provides patients the precise interventions they need, delivered properly, precisely when they need them. Fidelity is lacking when patients cannot make known their need for care (e.g., there are barriers in access or communication), when clinicians cannot recognize that an intervention is indicated (e.g., there is a lack of time, knowledge, attention, or memory), and when the intervention cannot be delivered properly (e.g., there is inadequate infrastructure, procedures, safety, coordination, or information). Fidelity has less to do with the properties of interventions than with the functionality of the system that delivers them. It requires systems of care (e.g., practice groups, hospitals) to have intelligent designs, skilled professionals, coordinated teams, adequate resources, competent information systems, reminders and other decision support tools, cooperation across organizations to achieve seamlessness, and a leadership culture committed to patient-centered care.[3-5] Assembling these conditions is one major way for society to improve the health of the population.

Efficacy and Effectiveness

The second strategy to alleviate disease is to enhance the *efficacy* (and effectiveness) of interventions. No treatment is perfect. Health can be improved if screening and diagnostic procedures are made more accurate and if treatments can perform better in reducing morbidity and mortality. This enterprise involves basic biomedical research; the translation from basic science to human application; and clinical trials to evaluate effectiveness, safety, adverse effects, and costs. The effort to improve efficacy and effectiveness involves the development of new agents and products in university-based and private industrial laboratories, and the dissemination of these products through licensing, advertising, and other channels. This prodigious technological investment to perfect new drugs and procedures is the second major way for society to improve the health of the population.

Society's Priorities

An objective observer would concede that the United States devotes most of its resources to the second aim, the enhancement of efficacy. The pharmaceutical industry spends $32 billion annually to develop new drugs and biologics.[6] This amount exceeds the entire $29 billion budget of the National Institutes of Health, which, in turn, spends most of its research dollars on basic science and translational research to bring new drugs and technologies to market.[7]

In contrast, our society spends relatively little on fidelity. Health systems spend greatly on delivering care – both on its administration and on competition for patients – but they spend relatively little on the important system redesigns that are essential to deliver care well. Although progressive institutions – exemplified by the Veterans Administration,[8] "breakthrough collaboratives,"[9,10] and leading health systems[11] – have enacted bold system redesigns and achieved notable success in delivering the right care at the right time, most health systems and private practices have moved less boldly.[12,13] Unlike the leaders of other industries who have committed themselves to quality, managers in health care have not embraced the need for system restructuring and have not committed resources to optimize service to their clients.[14] In addition, policy makers have not resolved the barriers to access and health insurance that deny care to at least 45 million Americans.[15]

Society's investment in research also includes little for fidelity. The annual budget of the federal agency with chief responsibility for this type of research, the Agency for Healthcare Research and Quality, is approximately $300 million, $1 for every $100 appropriated to the National Institutes of Health.[16] Private industry spends as much to develop just one new drug.[17,18] The spirit of inquiry and innovation that scientists apply to the creation of new technologies could yield ingenious solutions to the problems of health care delivery if similar levels of intellectual energy and financial resources were brought to bear.[19] Society's choice to channel billions of dollars into the race for new drugs and devices suggests that it values efficacy over fidelity as a priority for improvement.

Health Gains of Efficacy and Fidelity in Perspective

Is this strategy good for the population? The question is posed not to argue against the need for improving efficacy, which is vital, but rather to examine whether the balance is correct. The ethical principle of utilitarianism[20] compels a thoughtful examination of how efficacy and fidelity should be prioritized to accomplish the greatest good for the population's health (and the corollary, the extent to which imbalanced priorities contribute to disease).

Suppose a disease claims 100,000 lives each year and a drug is available that reduces the mortality rate from that disease by 20% (relative risk reduction [RRR] = 0.20). The drug therefore has the potential to save 20,000 lives each year, but if only 80% of eligible patients receive the drug, only 16,000 deaths will be averted (see Figure 1, A1). If society made no effort to improve the efficacy of the drug but managed to deliver it to 100% of eligible persons, 20,000 (4,000 additional) lives would be saved (*see* Figure 1, A2). But if society retains the 20% gap in delivery and works to enhance the efficacy of the drug, the RRR would have to rise above 25% ($100,000 \times 0.25 \times 0.8 = 20,000$), what we call the break-even point, to do as much good (i.e., to save 4,000 additional lives) (*see* Figure 1, A3).

The greater the gaps in delivery, the more efficacy must be increased to make that enterprise more beneficial than improving delivery, as shown in Figure 1. For example, if the assumptions in the above scenario are held constant, but 60%, rather than 80%, of the eligible population receives the medication, the RRR would have to rise from 20% to 33.3% to make the enhancement of drug efficacy more beneficial than improved delivery. When access to efficacious interventions is poor, large and unrealistic increases in efficacy must be achieved to surpass the potential gains from improving fidelity.

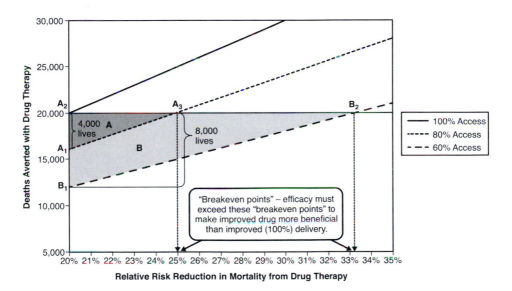

FIGURE 1 "The break-even point" (for a drug that reduces mortality by 20%)

Triangle A. If 100,000 patients are destined to die from a disease, a drug that reduces death rates by 20% (relative risk reduction [RRR] = 0.20) will save 16,000 lives (A1) if delivered to 80% of eligible patients. Increasing delivery to 100% would save 4,000 more lives (A2). To save as many lives with without improving upon the delivery rate of 80% (A3), the RRR of the drug must be increased to at least 25% ("break-even point").

Triangle B. Delivering the drug to only 60% of patients would save only 12,000 lives (B1), and improving delivery to 100% would save 8,000 additional lives. To save 8,000 additional lives without improving upon the delivery rate of 60% (B2), the RRR of the drug must be increased to at least 33.3% ("break-even point"). Developing a more efficacious drug is more beneficial than improving access only if the new relative risk reduction (RRR) exceeds the existing RRR divided by the proportion of the population exposed to treatment. The complete nomogram from which the figure derives is provided in Figure 2.

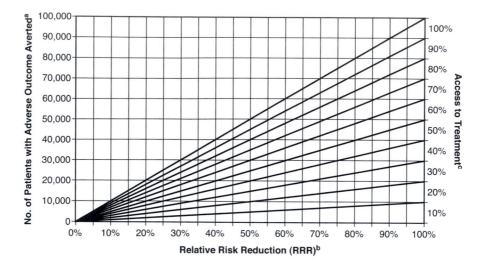

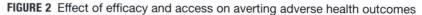

FIGURE 2 Effect of efficacy and access on averting adverse health outcomes

Note: The nomogram assumes a hypothetical population in which 100,000 patients are destined to experience an adverse health outcome (e.g., stroke, death). **a**. The number of patients in the cohort of 100,000 whose adverse outcome will be averted by treatment. **b**. The efficacy of a drug or other treatment in reducing the risk of the adverse outcome (eg, a relative risk reduction [RRR] = 0.40 means that the treatment will reduce the risk of the adverse outcome by a relative 40%). **c**. The proportion of the eligible patient population that receives the treatment. The nomogram shows that dramatic, often unrealistic, increases in RRR must be achieved to avert outcomes as effectively as improved access. To use the nomogram, select the RRR (**b**, x-axis) of a treatment and plot the location on the graph that corresponds with the frequency with which eligible patients receive the treatment (**c**, right-hand y-axis). The corresponding value on the left-hand y-axis (**a**) is the number of patients in the cohort of 100,000 whose adverse outcome will be averted. Move the plot vertically to a higher proportion with access (**c**) to determine how many more adverse outcomes (**a**) will be averted by improved delivery. From this location, move the plot horizontally to the right to determine how much RRR (**b**) must be increased to avert as many adverse outcomes. A specific example is provided in Figure 1 which enlarges a portion of this nomogram.

Is the Comparison Fair?

It might be argued that investments to enhance efficacy have a better track record of success than perfecting the delivery of care, making these hypothetical calculations unrealistic. Medicine can point to dramatic gains in improving efficacy, whereas the intractable barriers to achieving fidelity make the goal of 100% access seem untenable. But the assumptions underlying this argument deserve scrutiny.

First, although biotechnological research does yield stunning advances, the denominator is populated by a much larger number of failures. Only one of 10,000 compounds investigated by the pharmaceutical industry becomes a new drug. Only 20% of new drug applications to the Food and Drug Administration progress through clinical trials and are approved as new drugs.[17,18] Much biotech-nological research yields negative results or produces new agents or technologies of minimal value over standard care (e.g., "me-too" drugs). Only 22% of the drugs approved by the Food and Drug Administration represent "significant improve-ment compared with marketed products."[18] When stunning advances in efficacy are set against the denominator of all private and public research efforts, the net public health benefit from the endeavor is modest.

Second, the notion that fidelity cannot be markedly improved is mistaken. A large body of trial evidence suggests otherwise.[21] According to some reviews, the probability of providing the right care can be increased by as much as 68% through educational outreach and social marketing, 250% by offering feedback to clinicians about their performance, and 420% by instituting reminder systems.[22,23] Quality is improved and errors are reduced by building systems with integrated, multifaceted features that "make it hard for people to do the wrong thing."[24] Integrated system redesign, popularized by the work of Berwick[3] and Shortell et al,[25] is embodied in the Chronic Care Model and has improved outcomes for patients with chronic diseases.[26]

Large-scale system redesign has been recognized for some time as an urgent public health priority. Warning in 2001 that the health care system was funda-mentally flawed, a landmark Institute of Medicine report, *Crossing the Quality Chasm*, urged the nation and systems of care to undertake bold design changes to close the gap between what is and what should be done in health care.[24] The report called for major changes to create a system of care that was safe, effective, patient centered, timely, efficient, and equitable.

In the five years since that stark warning was issued, billions of dollars have flowed into the development of drugs and technologies, but a national resolve to rebuild systems to improve delivery is lacking. This imbalance in the priority given to efficacy vs fidelity has potentially serious consequences to population health, as the following two examples illustrate.

Antiplatelet Therapy to Prevent Recurrent Stroke

A systematic review by the Antithrombotic Trialists Collaboration[27] reported that the use of aspirin by patients who had previously experienced a stroke or transient ischemic attack reduces the incidence of recurrent nonfatal strokes by 23%. That is, in a population in which 100,000 people were destined to have strokes, 23,000 events could be prevented if all eligible patients took aspirin. McGlynn et al[1] reported, however, that antiplatelet therapy is given to only 58% of eligible patients. At that rate, only 13,340 strokes would be prevented in the hypothetical population, whereas achieving 100% fidelity in offering aspirin would prevent 23,000 strokes (i.e., 9,660 additional strokes).

Not addressing the fidelity of aspirin delivery and opting instead to develop better drugs makes sense (given the reasoning outlined above) only if the newer agents can lower stroke incidence by at least 40% (100,000 × 0.40 × 0.58 = 23, 000), but this increased efficacy would require a proportional improvement over aspirin of 74%. The pharmaceutical industry has invested heavily in alternative antiplatelet therapies; clopidogrel and ticlopidine underwent extensive testing in trials involving 22,976 subjects. Rather than demonstrating a 74% improvement over aspirin, however, these drugs were only 10% to 12% more effective in preventing vascular events.[27] It is worth asking whether the resources expended for the antiplatelet trials might have prevented more vascular events if they were invested in better systems for the delivery of aspirin.

Statin Use by Patients with Coronary Artery Disease

The use of simvastatin or pravastatin by patients with coronary artery disease reduces 5-year coronary artery disease mortality by as much as 24%.[28–30] McGlynn et al[1] report, however, that statins are prescribed to only 33% of eligible patients. Using the logic outlined above, we can posit that developing statins that surpass simvastatin or pravastatin is better for population health than achieving 100% uptake only if the new agents are three times as potent, reducing 5-year coronary artery disease mortality by at least 72% (100,000 × 0.72 × 0.33 = 24,000).

The degree to which the new generation of statins (e.g., atorvastatin, rosuvastatin) lower mortality is unknown, pending the results of ongoing trials, but the evidence regarding their effects on lipid levels suggests that they are not three times as potent. Rosuvastatin is only 26% more effective than pravastatin and 12% to 18% more effective than simvastatin in lowering levels of low-density lipoprotein cholesterol.[31] Although this superiority is clinically significant, we conclude that developing these agents has done less to save lives than would robust delivery systems that bring the older statins to all eligible patients.

That care processes can be modified to improve the delivery of cardiac drugs is hardly unrealistic.[32] Even simple interventions can have dramatic effects. One trial – conducted in a setting wherein 33% of patients with coronary artery disease were receiving lipid-lowering therapy – demonstrated the effectiveness of a simple reminder system: affixing a red notice to the front of the chart, citing current guidelines and the changes necessary to restore adherence.[33] Drug therapy was instituted or increased in 94% of patients in the intervention group but in only 10% of control patients, for whom no reminders were used.

Consider the choice of investing society's resources in making such reminder systems routine vs developing more potent drugs. If rosuvastatin is 26% more effective than pravastatin in lowering lipid levels,[31] we postulate (in the absence of direct evidence about mortality benefits) that the drug would reduce 5-year coronary artery disease mortality by an additional 6% (0.24 × 0.26), saving an additional 2,000 lives in our hypothetical population (100,000 × 0.06 × 0.33). In contrast, if older statins were retained but reminder systems were made routine, 14,640 additional lives might be saved (100,000 × 0.24 × [0.94 – 0.33]). In essence, forfeiting rosuvastatin to improve delivery of existing statins would have saved seven times as many lives (14,640/2,000).

Establishing reminder systems in the office of every physician in the nation would be costly, but developing new drugs is also exorbitant, with a cost of approximately $800 million per agent.[17] Spending on statins might be higher, given the size of the trials.[34] Even an investment of $800 million to develop a new statin would provide $28 for each of the estimated 28.4 million Americans[35] who ought to receive statins, a sum that could subsidize the cost of reminder systems for eligible patients.

Limitations

This thesis encounters problems at both the methodological and policy levels. The first methodological limitation is that relative risk rates and the estimates of proportion of the eligible population who receive recommended treatments are subject to error. The point estimates we used obscure the heterogeneity with which interventions perform across agents and settings. Second, the calculations assume that patients not receiving interventions face the same risk, and benefit equivalently, as those with access. Third, 100% uptake is rarely attainable, and the calculations should be adjusted for more realistic expectations. Formidable challenges impede the delivery of care to disadvantaged and minority populations, who are disproportionately affected by inadequate access and health insurance and by disparities in care.[2] Fourth, the hard endpoint of receipt of a service does not capture whether the service was delivered well, with quality, safety, and compassion.

Beyond its methodological limitations, our thesis encounters its greatest difficulties at the policy level. First, we pose a false dichotomy by suggesting that the pursuit of efficacy and fidelity are mutually exclusive, when one endeavor may enhance the other. For example, uptake of therapy can be improved if industry develops more acceptable products or if advertising campaigns alert patients and their clinicians to the need for treatment. A major reason why eligible patients do not take lipid-lowering medication – lack of awareness or agreement that the drugs are necessary[36] – may be mitigated by pharmaceutical companies' billion-dollar advertising campaigns.[37,38]

Second, this article focuses on investment in new products when often the trade-off involves the intensity of care. For example, while many women receive mammograms and Papanicolaou tests more frequently than needed,[39,40] 47% of eligible American Indian and Alaskan Native women have not had a recent mammogram.[41] Resources consumed by the overuse of care might do more good if deployed to serve those receiving inadequate care. Allocation of resources based on the relative effectiveness of health care services and the size of the population at risk (e.g., allocating for childhood immunizations vs heart transplantations) could further enhance population health.[42,43] A British study calculated that reducing cardiac risk factors had saved 731,720 life-years in England and Wales, compared with 194,145 life-years gained by cardiac treatments.[44]

Third, our analysis focuses only on selected health benefits of improving efficacy and fidelity. A fuller comparison would consider other health outcomes, harms, and costs, and would elucidate trade-offs in priority populations (e.g., racial and ethnic minorities, children, the elderly).[45]

Fourth and most important, the thesis envisions a nonexistent decision maker in American society, one who is responsible and controls resources for both technology development and systems to improve care delivery. In our health care system, private-sector manufacturers are largely responsible for allocating resources to drug and technology development, whereas managers of health systems and government agencies decide how much to spend on quality improvement. The wealth engine in private industry is not a resource shared with health plans to redesign systems of care.

Competing Agendas

It may be idealistic to expect decision makers in health systems or private industry to retain a global perspective – considering which strategy serves the greater good for the population – when other priorities influence their resource allocation decisions. Pharmaceutical companies care about population health but are also accountable to shareholders. Promoting statins is not just a public health exercise but also a $22 billion industry.[46] AstraZeneca's investment in rosuvastatin was an effort more to compete with Pfizer's atorvastatin than to meet a health need in the population.[47]

Capitalism and altruism can work at cross-purposes. A company faced with potential blockbuster earnings – such as the $2 to $3 billion per year that both clopidogrel and rosuvastatin generate[48] – is not expected to forgo its profits and donate its development budget to help health systems improve fidelity, potentially improving uptake of competitors' products, even if these campaigns will ultimately do more for population health.

Industry's technological advancement finds support with the American public, which marvels over scientific discovery and technological breakthroughs.[49] Robotic devices and genome mapping are more thrilling than bland quality improvement efforts, such as reminder systems and organizational redesign, irrespective of whether the latter saves more lives.[50]

The state is responsible for population health, but it can control only public budgets and cannot ensure that the vast and widely distributed resources of the health care system are deployed in rational proportions. Rarely are the complexities of health optimization first on the minds of government decision makers. Legislators and political appointees focus on pleasing constituents. Regulatory requirements, not health optimization, guide the choices of many agency officials. Neither the Food and Drug Administration nor the Centers for Medicare and Medicaid Services explicitly considers how the resources consumed by the interventions it approves compromise more effective strategies to improve public health.[51,52]

Although it may be appropriate to their work cultures for decision makers to base their choices on parochial concerns, the public ultimately suffers if, in the end, interventions that will do the most good are displaced by less beneficial measures. The ethic of utilitarianism[20] and the duty to provide care to all in need[53] create moral imperatives to design systems to ensure that care is delivered well to everyone. This imperative compels society to marshal the resources, intellectual energy, and national resolve for the reconfiguration of structure and process that excellence in care requires.[24]

Policy makers committed to fidelity would orchestrate the system solutions that expert panels[24,54] have recommended but that only selected health centers and communities have implemented.[55] They would establish universal health insurance,[15,56] remove financial barriers to care for the poor,[57] and address other causes of disparities.[2] They would transform today's visionary ideas for a new model of care[58] into tomorrow's reality. They would restructure delivery systems and realign reimbursement to promote the most effective treatments and to replace current fragmentation with seamless delivery.[9,25] They would provide open access,[59] e-mail consultations,[60] and other innovations to ensure timely assistance and fewer errors. They would invest in information systems to connect patients with the finest educational resources, decision aids, and electronic health records.[61,62] Communities would build integrated linkages between health care professionals and civic partners – for example, work sites, schools, and churches – to help patients implement medical advice after they leave the clinic.[25,63]

The future may bring greater public interest in fidelity as frustration with health care deepens.[64] A national survey found that 55% of Americans were dissatisfied with the quality of health care in 2004, up from 44% in 2000.[65] In time, the public may come to view new technological wizardry as less of a "medical advance" than provision of prompt clinical attention; responsiveness; preventive services; skilled care that is coordinated, evidence based, and error free; timely reminders; clear communication; immediate access to information; cultural sensitivity; equity; and respect.[2,9,25,59,62,66–74]

That private and public leaders have chosen instead to invest comparatively little in achieving these aims and to commit the bulk of resources to making better treatments for those who receive care is not only problematic in terms of equity, but, as we have shown, a potential contributor to excess deaths and morbidity. Both lives and ethics are thus at stake.

Individual physicians can press their leaders, both civic and professional, to make fidelity a higher priority,[75] and they can promote fidelity in daily practice. This article shows that prescribing the latest drug may help patients less than adopting office systems to ensure that all eligible individuals receive recommended care.[76] Clinicians should look past catchy drug advertisements and the promotions of pharmaceutical representatives to consider whether the incremental magnitude of benefit offered by newer agents crosses the break-even point (*see* Figure 1).

As a society, we should confront the price we pay – in human lives – by maintaining a health care system that is not designed to deliver care well. Society can realign its priorities. It can spend less profligately on the enhancement of drugs and technology, and redesign systems of care to ensure a standard of excellence that fulfills the attributes of quality outlined in the *Chasm* report[24] and the Future of Family Medicine project.[58] Failure to act to correct deficiencies in fidelity is, in effect, an affirmative choice to subject patients to greater illness and suffering. To do so while investing vast wealth in technology should weigh heavily on society's collective conscience.

References

1. McGlynn EA, Asch SM, Adams J, et al. The quality of health care delivered to adults in the United States. *N Engl J Med.* 2003; 348: 2635–45.
2. Smedley BD, Stith AY, Nelson AR, eds. Committee on Understanding and Eliminating Racial and Ethnic Disparities in Health Care BoHSP, Institute of Medicine. *Unequal Treatment: Confronting Racial and Ethnic Disparities in Health Care.* Washington, DC: National Academies Press; 2003.
3. Berwick DM. A primer on leading the improvement of systems. *BMJ.* 1996; 312: 619–22.
4. Von Korff M, Gruman J, Schaefer J, Curry SJ, Wagner EH. Collaborative management of chronic illness. *Ann Intern Med.* 1997; 127: 1097–1102.
5. Berwick DM. Improvement, trust, and the healthcare workforce. *Qual Saf Health Care.* 2003; 12: 448–52.
6. Pharmaceutical Research and Manufacturers of America. Washington, DC. *Pharmaceutical R&D spending: PhRMA Annual Membership Survey, 2002.* 2002. Available at: www.phrma.org/issues/research-dev/ (accessed October 8, 2003).
7. Sung NS, Crowley WF Jr, Genel M, et al. Central challenges facing the national clinical research enterprise. *JAMA.* 2003; 289: 1278–87.
8. Jha AK, Perlin JB, Kizer KW, Dudley RA. Effect of the transformation of the Veterans Affairs Health Care System on the quality of care. *N Engl J Med.* 2003; 348: 2218–27.
9. Wagner EH, Glasgow RE, Davis C, et al. Quality improvement in chronic illness care: a collaborative approach. *Jt Comm J Qual Improv.* 2001; 27: 63–80.
10. Berwick D, Rothman M. Pursuing perfection: an interview with Don Berwick and Michael Rothman. Interview by Andrea Kabcenell and Jane Roessner. *Jt Comm J Qual Improv.* 2002; 28: 268–78, 209.
11. Solberg LI, Hroscikoski MC, Sperl-Hillen JM, O'Connor PJ, Crabtree BF. Key issues in transforming health care organizations for quality: the case of advanced access. *Jt Comm J Qual Saf.* 2004; 30: 15–24.
12. Becher EC, Chassin MR. Improving the quality of health care: who will lead? *Health Aff (Millwood).* 2001; 20: 164–79.
13. Berwick DM. Disseminating innovations in health care. *JAMA.* 2003; 289: 1969–75.
14. Chassin MR. Is health care ready for Six Sigma quality? *Milbank Q.* 1998; 76: 565–91, 510.
15. Committee on the Consequences of Uninsurance, Board on Health Care Services, Institute of Medicine. *Care Without Coverage: Too Little, Too Late.* Washington, DC: National Academy Press; 2002.
16. Clancy CM. AHRQ's FY 2005 budget request: new mission, new vision. *Health Serv Res.* 2004; 39: xi–xviii.
17. DiMasi JA, Hansen RW, Grabowski HG. The price of innovation: new estimates of drug development costs. *J Health Econ.* 2003; 22: 151–85.
18. Public Citizen. *Rx R&D Myths: The Case Against The Drug Industry's R&D "Scare Card."* 2001. Available at: www.citizen.org/publications/release.cfm?ID=7065.
19. Berwick DM. Crossing the boundary: changing mental models in the service of improvement. *Int J Qual Health Care.* 1998; 10: 435–41.
20. Gillon R. Utilitarianism. *Br Med J (Clin Res Ed).* 1985; 290: 1411–13.
21. Agency for Healthcare and Research Quality. *Translating Research Into Practice (TRIP)-II. Fact sheet.* Rockville, Md: AHRQ; 2001. Available at: www.ahrq.gov/research/trip2fac.htm.
22. Thomson O'Brien MA, Oxman AD, Davis DA, et al. Educational outreach visits: effects on professional practice and health care outcomes. *Cochrane Database Syst Rev.* 2000: CD000409.
23. Bennett JW, Glasziou PP. Computerised reminders and feedback in medication management: a systematic review of randomised controlled trials. *Med J Aust.* 2003; 178: 217–22.

24. Committee on Quality of Health Care in America, Institute of Medicine. *Crossing the Quality Chasm: A New Health System for the 21st Century.* Washington, DC: National Academy Press; 2001.

25. Shortell SM, Gillies RR, Anderson DA. *Remaking Health Care in America.* 2nd ed. San Francisco, CA: Jossey-Bass; 2000.

26. Bodenheimer T, Wagner EH, Grumbach K. Improving primary care for patients with chronic illness. *JAMA.* 2002; 288: 1775–79.

27. Collaborative meta-analysis of randomised trials of antiplatelet therapy for prevention of death, myocardial infarction, and stroke in high risk patients. *BMJ.* 2002; 324: 71–86.

28. MRC/BHF Heart Protection Study of cholesterol lowering with simvastatin in 20,536 high-risk individuals: a randomised placebo-controlled trial. *Lancet.* 2002; 360: 7–22.

29. Sacks FM, Pfeffer MA, Moye LA, et al. The effect of pravastatin on coronary events after myocardial infarction in patients with average cholesterol levels. Cholesterol and Recurrent Events Trial investigators. *N Engl J Med.* 1996; 335: 1001–09.

30. Prevention of cardiovascular events and death with pravastatin in patients with coronary heart disease and a broad range of initial cholesterol levels. The Long-Term Intervention with Pravastatin in Ischaemic Disease (LIPID) Study Group. *N Engl J Med.* 1998; 339: 1349–57.

31. Jones PH, Davidson MH, Stein EA, et al. Comparison of the efficacy and safety of rosuvastatin versus atorvastatin, simvastatin, and pravastatin across doses (STELLAR* Trial). *Am J Cardiol.* 2003; 92: 152–60.

32. Miller NH, Hill M, Kottke T, Ockene IS. The multilevel compliance challenge: recommendations for a call to action. A statement for healthcare professionals. *Circulation.* 1997; 95: 1085–90.

33. Stamos TD, Shaltoni H, Girard SA, Parrillo JE, Calvin JE. Effectiveness of chart prompts to improve physician compliance with the National Cholesterol Education Program guidelines. *Am J Cardiol.* 2001; 88: 1420–23, A1428.

34. McKillop T. The statin wars [letter]. *Lancet.* 2003; 362: 1498.

35. Jacobson TA, Griffiths GG, Varas C, et al. Impact of evidence-based "clinical judgment" on the number of American adults requiring lipid-lowering therapy based on updated NHANES III data. National Health and Nutrition Examination Survey. *Arch Intern Med.* 2000; 160: 1361–69.

36. Pearson TA, Feinberg W. Behavioral issues in the efficacy versus effectiveness of pharmacologic agents in the prevention of cardiovascular disease. *Ann Behav Med.* 1997; 19: 230–38.

37. Noonan D. You want statins with that? *Newsweek.* July 14, 2003: 34–48.

38. Barnett M. Pill profits. *US News and World Report.* December 22, 2003; 135: 40.

39. Kerlikowske K, Smith-Bindman R, Sickles EA. Short-interval follow-up mammography: are we doing the right thing? *J Natl Cancer Inst.* 2003; 95: 418–19.

40. Ostbye T, Greenberg GN, Taylor DH Jr, Lee AM. Screening mammography and Pap tests among older American women 1996–2000: results from the Health and Retirement Study (HRS) and Asset and Health Dynamics Among the Oldest Old (AHEAD). *Ann Fam Med.* 2003; 1: 209–17.

41. National Center for Health Statistics. *Health, United States, 2003 With Chartbook on Trends in the Health of Americans.* Hyattsville, Md: 2003. Available at: www.cdc.gov/nchs/data/hus/hus03.pdf.

42. Murray CJL, Evans DB, eds. *Health Systems Performance Assessment: Debates, Methods and Empiricism.* Geneva, Switzerland: World Health Organization; 2003.

43. Stevens A, Raftery J, eds. *Health Care Needs Assessment.* Oxford: Radcliffe Medical Press; 1997.

44. Unal B, Critchley JA, Fidan D, Capewell S. Life-years gained from modern cardiological treatments and population risk factor changes in England and Wales, 1981–2000. *Am J Public Health.* 2005; 95: 103–08.

45. Leatherman S, Berwick D, Iles D, et al. The business case for quality: case studies and an analysis. *Health Aff (Millwood)*. 2003; 22: 17–30.

46. Herper M. Statin makers bet big on imaging technique. *Forbes*. November 10, 2003. Available at: www.forbes.com/2003/11/10/cx_mh_1110merck.html (accessed July 30, 2012).

47. Barrett A, Carey J. A bare knuckle battle over cholesterol drugs. *Business Week*. July 21, 2003: 28.

48. Foster G. Bears sink teeth into AstraZeneca. *This Is London*. November 11, 2003. Available at: www.standard.co.uk/news/bears-sink-teeth-into-astrazeneca-6975937.html (accessed July 30, 2012).

49. Hospitalnetwork.com. *HIMA 2000: Manufacturers Updated on Medicare Reform, Healthcare Policy. The Politics of Healthcare Policy*. Available at: www.hospitalnetwork.com/doc.mvc/HIMA-2000-Manufacturers-Updated-on-Medicare-R-0001#the (accessed July 30, 2012).

50. Milstein A, Adler NE. Out of sight, out of mind: why doesn't widespread clinical quality failure command our attention? *Health Aff (Millwood)*. 2003; 22: 119–27.

51. Medicare program: Negotiated rulemaking: Coverage and administrative policies for clinical diagnostic laboratory services; final rule. CFR 42 66: 410: 58788–58836. Available at: www.cms.gov/Medicare/Coverage/CoverageGenInfo/Downloads/lab1.pdf.

52. Meadows M. The FDA's drug review process: ensuring drugs are safe and effective. *FDA Consumer Magazine*. July–August 2002. FDA publication No. 02–3242.

53. Smith R, Hiatt H, Berwick D. Shared ethical principles for everybody in health care: a working draft from the Tavistock group. *BMJ*. 1999; 318: 248–51.

54. Adams K, Corrigan JM, eds. Committee on Identifying Priority Areas for Quality Improvement. Board on Health Care Services, Institute of Medicine. *Priority Areas for National Action: Transforming Health Care Quality*. Washington, DC: National Academies Press; 2003.

55. Corrigan JM, Greiner A, Erickson SM, eds. Committee on Rapid Advance Demonstration Projects: Health Care Finance and Delivery Systems, Institute of Medicine. *Fostering Rapid Advances in Health Care: Learning from System Demonstrations*. Washington, DC: National Academies Press; 2002.

56. Committee on the Consequences of Uninsurance, Board on Health Care Services, Institute of Medicine. *Insuring America's Health: Principles and Recommendations*. Washington, DC: National Academies Press; 2004.

57. Himmelstein DU, Warren E, Thorne D, Woolhandler S. MarketWatch: Illness and injury as contributors to bankruptcy. *Health Aff (Millwood)*. February 2, 2005 [Web exclusive]. Available at: http://content.healthaffairs.org/cgi/reprint/hlthaff.w5.63v1 (accessed September 6, 2005).

58. Martin JC, Avant RF, Bowman MA, et al. The future of family medicine: a collaborative project of the family medicine community. *Ann Fam Med*. 2004; 2(Suppl 1): S3–S32.

59. Murray M, Bodenheimer T, Rittenhouse D, Grumbach K. Improving timely access to primary care: case studies of the advanced access model. *JAMA*. 2003; 289: 1042–46.

60. Car J, Sheikh A. Email consultations in health care: 1 – scope and effectiveness. *BMJ*. 2004; 329: 435–38.

61. Bodenheimer T, Grumbach K. Electronic technology: a spark to revitalize primary care? *JAMA*. 2003; 290: 259–64.

62. Glasgow RE, Bull SS, Piette JD, Steiner JF. Interactive behavior change technology: a partial solution to the competing demands of primary care. *Am J Prev Med*. 2004; 27: 80–87.

63. Safran DG. Defining the future of primary care: what can we learn from patients? *Ann Intern Med*. 2003; 138: 248–55.

64. Murphy J, Chang H, Montgomery JE, Rogers WH, Safran DG. The quality of physician-patient relationships: patients' experiences 1996–1999. *J Fam Pract*. 2001; 50: 123–29.

65. The Kaiser Family Foundation/Agency for Healthcare Research and Quality/Harvard School of Public Health. *National Survey on Consumers' Experiences With Patient Safety and Quality Information*. Washington, DC: Henry J. Kaiser Family Foundation; 2004. Publication No. 7209.

66. Kuzel AJ, Woolf SH, Gilchrist VJ, et al. Patient reports of preventable problems and harms in primary health care. *Ann Fam Med*. 2004; 2: 333–40.
67. Coffield AB, Maciosek MV, McGinnis JM, et al. Priorities among recommended clinical preventive services. *Am J Prev Med*. 2001; 21: 1–9.
68. Woolf SH, George JN. Evidence-based medicine: interpreting studies and setting policy. *Hematol Oncol Clin North Am*. 2000; 14: 761–84.
69. Kohn LT, Corrigan JM, Donaldson MS, eds. Committee on Quality of Health Care in America, Institute of Medicine. *To Err is Human: Building a Safer Health System*. Washington, DC: National Academies Press; 2000.
70. Szilagyi PG, Bordley C, Vann JC, et al. Effect of patient reminder/recall interventions on immunization rates: a review. *JAMA*. 2000; 284: 1820–27.
71. Schmittdiel J, McMenamin SB, Halpin HA, et al. The use of patient and physician reminders for preventive services: results from a National Study of Physician Organizations. *Prev Med*. 2004; 39: 1000–06.
72. Nielsen-Bohlman L, Panzer AM, Kindig DA, eds. Committee on Health Literacy, Board on Neuroscience and Behavioral Health, Institute of Medicine. *Health Literacy: A Prescription to End Confusion*. Washington, DC: National Academies Press; 2004.
73. Committee on Communication for Behavior Change in the 21st Century: Improving the Health of Diverse Populations, Board on Neuroscience and Behavioral Health, Institute of Medicine. *Speaking of Health: Assessing Health Communication Strategies for Diverse Populations*. Washington, DC: National Academies Press; 2002.
74. Gallagher A. Dignity and respect for dignity – two key health professional values: implications for nursing practice. *Nurs Ethics*. 2004; 11: 587–99.
75. Gruen RL, Pearson SD, Brennan TA. Physician-citizens – public roles and professional obligations. *JAMA*. 2004; 291: 94–98.
76. Dickey LL, Gemson DH, Carney P. Office system interventions supporting primary care-based health behavior change counseling. *Am J Prev Med*. 1999; 17: 299–308.

40

Ecological Change and the Future of the Human Species

Can Physicians Make a Difference?

Roger A. Rosenblatt, MD, MPH, MFR

Case Report

The patient is an elderly woman, beloved in her community, who comes to your office with a list of serious problems. She has night sweats and fevers that have been getting worse for the last few years. She has difficulty breathing and on examination seems to have suffered from aspiration pneumonia. She has alopecia, having lost her hair in a patchy distribution. Her normal gastrointestinal flora has been invaded by a few noxious species, and she has persistent diarrhea. Her skin is marked by an extensive dermatitis: it is fissured, inflamed, gouged, scraped, denuded, and cracking in many places. These excoriations are caused by a small but extremely industrious organism whose numbers have grown exponentially during the last few years, displacing and even eliminating other organisms that used to be widely distributed on the skin of our patient (*see* Figure 1).

Differential Diagnosis: Global Environmental Change

The patient, of course, is Earth. Each symptom reflects one of a series of environmental perturbations that are threatening the homeostasis of the marvelous planet we call home.[1] It is useful to consider each of these symptoms individually and to examine the way they interact to spawn a disease complex that demands our urgent attention as physicians, humans, and members of a biological community.

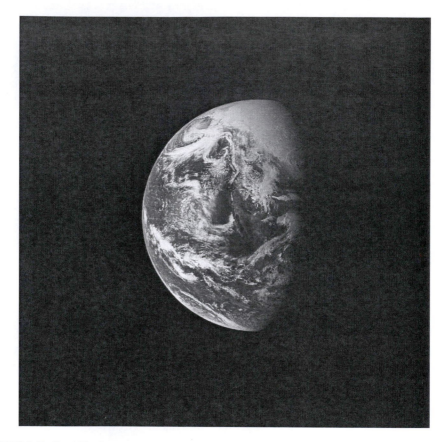

FIGURE 1 Patient Earth

Earth taken from Apollo 13, April 17, 1970. Source: NASA.

Night Sweats and Fevers: Global Warming

Human production of greenhouse gases – in particular carbon dioxide, methane, and the chlorofluorocarbons – has led to increases in Earth's surface temperature.[2] Global warming is a reality, and the inevitable rise in carbon dioxide alone will lead to further increases in mean global temperature of 2°F to 10°F this century. The problem is even more acute in the growing number of mega-cities in which the human population increasingly clusters.[3] These population centers become heat islands that are 7°F to 10°F hotter than the surrounding countryside.

The consequences of global warming will have profound effects on Earth and its inhabitants. Rising sea levels will cause flooding of low-lying islands and coastal communities.[4] Heat itself causes devastating heat waves. The 2003 summer heat wave in France killed 10 times more people than died from severe acute respiratory syndrome (SARS) worldwide between 2002 and 2004.[5,6] This climate change is very likely to increase the range of insect vectors that carry a number of virulent diseases, including malaria, dengue fever, West Nile virus, and encephalitis.[7]

The greatest culprit is the burning of fossil fuels to run our cars, factories, and the air conditioners with which we attempt to survive the heat waves that cause these global night sweats. As the developing world strives to match the lifestyles of the Western world, the problem will accelerate.

Respiratory Distress: Poor Air Quality

We take air for granted – usually. Breathe in, breathe out, thousands of times a day, millions of times in a lifetime. But breathing can be misery, and for growing numbers of people, respiration is a constant grim challenge.

Asthma is among the most common afflictions, and both the prevalence and the severity of this disease are increasing. Despite the development of powerful new treatments for asthma, wheezing kids fill our urban emergency departments. Epidemics of asthma sweep through urban communities with the rapidity and morbidity of influenza, but immunizations cannot protect the vulnerable.[9]

Although we do not fully understand all the elements of the respiratory disease epidemic that has swept the world during the last few decades, one factor is contaminated air.[7] The Clean Air Act of 1970 led to some improvements in air quality in the United States, but progress has not been uniform, and the administration of George W. Bush has attempted to weaken existing environmental protections.[9] Global warming exacerbates the impact of air pollution; ozone levels rise in tandem with air temperature, and ozone is one of the more virulent causes of air pollution.[7,8]

As we spew pollutants into the great common air sheds upon which we depend, everybody inhales equal opportunity toxins. Deteriorating air is further paralleled in polluted water, another rate-limiting substance upon which not only humans, but all species, depend.

Alopecia: Deforestation

Our patient's alopecia is mirrored in the deforestation of our globe. In the Amazon, forests are burned to allow crops to be planted, even though the thin soil is depleted after one or two crop rotations. In Nepal and Central America, growing rural populations walk farther each day from their villages to cut firewood from the dwindling forests. In Africa, drought and global warming feed the expanding deserts. In the 1990s alone, human activities led to the loss of more than 500,000 square miles of forests.[10]

The story of Easter Island illustrates how much our well-being is tied to the trees that support our world in more than a metaphoric way. Polynesians colonized the island in the fifth century, attracted in part by existing forests that seemed to offer an inexhaustible supply of wood to build houses, sea-going canoes, and the log rollers that allowed them to construct the fantastic stone monuments for which the island is famous.[11] The entire civilization collapsed several generations later largely because the trees were harvested unsustainably, leading to mass famine when the Easter islanders could not replace the canoes upon which their fishery depended.[12] The Polynesians who cut the trees did not imagine the catastrophic consequences of deforestation for their once-thriving civilization. Can we?

Diarrhea: Loss of Biodiversity

Just as our gastrointestinal tracts need a spectrum of normal bacteria for healthy functioning, our globe benefits from the amazing diversity of life. Evolution is beginning to run in reverse. Species that inhabited Earth long before humans emerged are being eradicated by mass extinctions.[13] As we crowd out other species by our manipulation of the globe, we are impoverished by the loss of species that provide us with food, oxygen, medicine, and aesthetic enjoyment.

Species extinction is invisible to most of us. The planetary system seems so robust that it seems unlikely that we could be threatened by the loss of a few bugs or birds that few of us have heard of. The whole intricate complex is quite fragile, however, and our genomic sciences are no substitute for the immense archive of DNA that is the legacy of billions of years of evolution. Which is the keystone species whose loss will lead to the collapse of the whole edifice?

Dermatitis: Overpopulation

The world's population has grown from fewer than 100 million people 3,000 years ago to 6.3 billion people today, with two thirds of the increase in the last 50 years.[10] By the year 2050 the world population is projected to range from 7.4 billion to 10.6 billion people.[14] The rapid growth in human population, and the increased resource consumption generated both by the sheer number of humans and the rapid pace of development has transformed Earth and altered the basic geochemical cycles upon which life depends.[15]

Although it may seem demeaning to think of the human species as a form of lice, our collective impact on the surface of the globe is even greater than that of scabies on the skin of our hapless patient. The human population has not only affected Earth's crust and the thin organic layer that covers it, but human activities have also depleted and polluted ground water, altered the chemistry of the atmosphere, and changed the genetic composition of much of the plant life growing on the planet.[16,17] The population burden of humans affects our own species as well as those with whom we share the globe.

Overpopulation not only drives environmental degradation but can contribute to poverty, social polarization, and large-scale human migration. Stabilization of Earth's human population is an important first step in any attempt to restore equilibrium to our natural and social processes.

The Medical Response: What Can We Do?

As Paul Ehrlich has pointed out, the human species is superb at countering acute crises and dismal at addressing slow-moving threats.[18] We have mobilized a rapid and effective global response to the threats represented by bioterrorism and SARS, but we seem paralyzed in the face of the much slower collapse of the ecosystem on which all depend.

Despair is unacceptable – the situation is much too serious for acquiescence. There are some concrete steps that we as citizens and health professionals can take.[19]

Expand Your Perspective

Just as we have gone beyond the purely biological in medicine to incorporate both the psychological and the social, so can we realize that there is an ecological dimension to much of what we do. We are related to all the other species carrying shards of billion-year-old DNA in their cells, and we share a common existence and a common fate. By increasing our awareness of the connectedness of all living organisms, we can use our talents as healers to restore the vitality of the web of life.

Help Prevent Unwanted Pregnancies

Probably the most important thing we can do as physicians is to help people control their own fertility. The most logical place to begin for those of us in family medicine would be in the area of family planning, an area in which we already have the clinical responsibility and the requisite skills. One of the most effective ways to stabilize population levels is to prevent unintended pregnancy.

The Wonder and the Mystery

A distressingly large proportion of pregnancies are unplanned and unwanted, often disrupting and impoverishing the families where they occur. Simply by reducing the number of unintended pregnancies, we could achieve a dramatic reduction in the overall birth rate, a reduction that if replicated worldwide could have a marked impact on the rate of population rise. Even though much of the problem lies outside the industrialized world, the United States has a disproportionate effect on the policies of other countries.

Encourage Sustainable Economies

We can use our influence to shape the economic activities of our own community, and change our own behavior to set an example. Economic development is critical to the social well-being of a community, but not if it destroys the resources on which it depends.[20]

Stay Engaged with the Natural World

Life is not a pixilated image on a shimmering screen. We must immerse ourselves in the exhilarating symphony of the natural world – cherish and preserve the beauty that remains, work to repair the damage done by others, and walk gently on this Earth.

The doctor is sanctioned by society as a healer and, as such, has the opportunity to influence the conditions that promote or undermine good health. This position of privilege also carries the responsibility to use our talents and energy, not only to mend the ills of our individual patients, but to improve the milieu in which they live. It is time to acknowledge the enormous ecological issues that affect the very substrate of life itself but that lie outside the traditional boundaries of our profession. The practice of medicine cannot proceed in a vacuum, insulated from the catastrophic changes in the ecosystem upon which life depends. We have the ability to repair much of the harm we have done. Now we need the will.

References

1. McMichael AJ. Global environmental change and human population health: a conceptual and scientific challenge for epidemiology. *Int J Epidemiol.* 1998; 221: 1–8.
2. *Intergovernmental Panel on Climate Change. Third Assessment Report, Vol. 1.* Cambridge: Cambridge University Press; 2001.
3. National Research Council. *Our Common Journey: A Transition Towards Sustainability.* Washington, DC: National Academy Press; 1999.
4. Tibbets J. Coastal cities: living on the edge. *Environ Health Perspect.* 2002; 20: 674–81.

5. Leicester J. France says 11,435 people died in heat wave. *The Detroit News.* August 30, 2004.
6. Summary of probable SARS cases with onset of illness from 1 November 2002 to 31 July 2003. WHO, Communicable Disease Surveillance and Response, 2004.
7. Haines A, Patz JA. Health effects of climate change. *JAMA.* 2004; 291: 99–103.
8. Thurston GD, Ito K. Epidemiological studies of acute ozone exposure and mortality. *J Expo Ann Environ Epidemiol.* 2001; 11: 286–94.
9. Paralysis on clean air [editorial]. *New York Times,* January 4, 2004: 6.
10. De Souza R, Williams JS, Meyerson FAB. Critical links: population, health and the environment. *Pop Bull.* 2003; 58: 1–44.
11. Chu EW, Karr JR. Environmental impact, concept and measurement. In: *Encyclopedia of Biodiversity, Volume 2.* Washington, DC: Academic Press; 2001.
12. Rees W. Revisiting carrying capacity: area-based indicators of sustainability. *Popul Environ.* 1996; 17: 195–215.
13. Wilson EO. *The Future of Life.* London: Little, Brown; 2002.
14. United Nations (UN) Population Division, World Population Prospects: The 2002 Revision. New York, NY: United Nations; 2003.
15. McMichael AJ, Powles JW. Human numbers, environment, sustainability, and health. *BMJ.* 1999; 319: 977–80.
16. Ehrlich PR, Ehrlich AH, Daily GC. Food security: population and environment. *Pop Devel Rev.* 1993; 19: 1–31.
17. Moomaw WR, Tullis MD. Population, affluence or technology? An empirical look at carbon dioxide production. In: Baudot B, Moomaw WR, eds. *People and Their Planet, Searching for Balance.* New York, NY: Palgrave Macmillan; 1999.
18. Ehrlich PR, Ehrlich AH. *Healing the Planet.* New York, NY: Addison-Wesley Publishing Company; 1991.
19. Gruen RL, Pearson SD, Brennan TA. Physician-citizens – public roles and professional obligations. *JAMA.* 2004; 294: 94–98.
20. Madden CW. Health care policy, economics, and ecological health. *Illahee.* 1994; 10: 114–18.

41

A Journey to Someplace Better

John J. Frey III, MD

OUR PRACTICE IS ONE OF TWO IN A COMMUNITY WHERE MANY OF US speak Spanish. The data from the 2000 census showed a 500% increase in the Hispanic population in our county. Some days it seems as though most of them find their way to our practice. One census map shows the counties in the United States with Latino populations of higher than 20%, and other than the obvious border counties of the Southwest and such places as Florida and New York, counties with large Latino populations are scattered right across the Great Plains from Ohio to Kansas and, in recent years, down into the Middle Atlantic states. Fluency in Spanish is more than a nice addition to a residency applicant's curriculum vitae; it gets extra points come time for the match.

Many young men whose jobs entail heavy manual labor in our county come to see me, and young women working in laundries and cleaning services see my female partners. The children see us all, accompanied by whoever is at home and able to take them to the doctor for illness visits or checkups. The staff has been at the clinic for decades and, in response to our changing population, has made valiant but frustrating attempts to learn basic Spanish. We all struggle to find words for bowel movements, impotence, anxiety, and depression that are not in the Spanish textbooks. I am forever running to find my partner who grew up in Mexico, asking her about words in Spanish I cannot seem to find or my patients do not seem to understand. She always smiles and shakes her head a bit when she tells me the correct way to phrase things.

During a busy clinic morning, I glanced at my schedule and saw names of patients I did not recognize, one of whom was a 9-year-old girl for a well-child examination for school. Because it was early summer, I assumed that she was just getting her checkup early to avoid the end-of-summer rush. Her name was Carolina.

I came into the examination room and saw her sitting in the chair next to her mother, a pleasant woman whom I had never met either. Carolina was sitting in a way that immediately caught my eye – like the little girl in a Norman Rockwell painting – long dress, hands folded together on her knees, her back upright against the back of the chair, making direct eye contact with me, a smile on her face. She seemed happy to be there, not the case with most 9-year-olds dragged by a parent to the clinic for a camp or school physical examination. (I have seen bemused interest on their faces, but not delight.) Her mother, after a quick glance at me and a polite hello, turned to look at Carolina with a glance almost of adoration. As I started asking questions, Carolina gave me most of the answers, except, of course, her early childhood illnesses. "I am here to get permission to go to school," she said. "She needs to get the vaccinations," her mother filled in. In addition to her immunizations, she needed some dental work, needed to eat a bit better, and had a long way to go to learn English.

"Well, where are you going to school," I asked. "I don't know," she answered, "I just arrived here." I asked her mother when they had come to the United States, and her mother said that she had been here two years, but that Carolina came last week.

"How did you get here?" I inquired, attempting to make small talk. "I came in the van," she answered, "last month, from Mexico, from my home in Morelos. I left our home town and went on a van to Mexico City, where I stayed for a while with some people, then we got on a bus and drove for a long time. When we got to a town, some of the people left for the mountains, and all of the rest of us stayed in a big room where there were police. After a while, they let me go and I got on another van and we came into the United States to a very big city. Then I got on another van and came here to be with my parents."

"Who did you come with?" I asked. "I came by myself, in the van with some other people," she replied. She smiled and looked at her mother, who in turn continued to gaze, lovingly, at her daughter. Nine years old, more than 3,000 miles, by herself.

I have learned from my patients during these years in practice that many men, mostly by themselves, but at other times with their wives, leave rural Mexico for places like our community because the word has gotten back to their hometowns that there are opportunities here for jobs. I always imagine signs in little towns scattered throughout Mexico and Central America that read, "Good jobs in

Madison" (or Dodge City or Cedar Rapids or Springfield), with a contact and a telephone number that starts someone thinking, "I could go there and do better."

The jobs make it possible to send money home to help improve the lives of their families, a story much like that of other groups which populated the history of our part of America. The names of little towns throughout Wisconsin proclaim which immigrant group settled there first – New Lisbon, New London, New Holstein, New Berlin, Germantown, Wales, Belgium. After the couples from Morelos or Oaxaca or Puebla feel that their jobs and lives are secure, they bring their children from Mexico. In bringing them, parents separate their children not only from friends and family but from all the familiar things of their children's lives and culture. The parents believe that, after a while, life will be better here and that their children will recover from the grief of lost homelands, will find friends, schools, a life. For the parents, the alternative of having their children raised 3,000 miles away by relatives is too much to bear. They need the reasons they work two jobs and live in small apartments right in front of their eyes to help them keep going.

I knew why Carolina's mother looked at her with such love. Her parents must have been frantic with fear, worrying and listening for her progress through towns and across borders, and then feeling the elation as she, the reason for their two jobs and long days, arrived in town. Ships sink, vans crash, people get arrested, get quarantined, get locked and smothered in trucks, or die of starvation. Sometimes they make it. Carolina's persistence in the face of such danger might have been because she was a child, too inexperienced to know any better. But I would like to believe it could also be her courage, trusting that her family sent her on a journey to someplace better, ignoring the evil that can, at times, seem to be everywhere, having faith that someone would care for her. Now she was here, safe, with her family, seeing a doctor, and getting ready for the next adventure.

The times here, too, are hard and getting harder. William Carlos Williams called the 1930s "the knife of the times that kills men's souls," and just under the surface of our patients' lives, that knife is pressing. Jobs are fewer and more demanding. Joblessness is real and growing, even in seemingly recession-proof cities like Madison. I worry that Carolina's family will be forced to make the long trip back to Morelos out of necessity rather than choice. I would be robbed of her presence, and I need it. When my world, on occasion, seems full of patients and friends who feel hopeless and too tired to continue, I imagine Carolina, hands firmly on her knees, riding a van, looking out the window at a world she has never seen toward a place she could only imagine. It is the image I need to make it through days when, sometimes, it feels as if all I see is despair – a solitary

9-year-old girl, full of hope and dreams, with a belief in guardian angels and in friendly, rather than threatening, strangers.

I asked Carolina what she was going to do after she went home. "Get ready," she said. "Next week I go to school."

Index